Pain
ITS NAT

Pain

ITS NATURE, ANALYSIS AND TREATMENT

Michael R. Bond
MD PhD FRCP(Glas) FRCS(Edin), FRCPsych
Professor of Psychological Medicine, University of Glasgow.
Department of Psychological Medicine, 6 Whittinghame Gardens,
Great Western Road, Glasgow.

FOREWORD BY

John J. Bonica
MD DSc FFARCS
Professor and Former Chairman, Deparment of Anaesthesiology, Director,
Pain Center, University of Washington School of Medicine, Seattle,
USA

SECOND EDITION

CHURCHILL LIVINGSTONE
EDINBURGH LONDON MELBOURNE AND NEW YORK 1984

CHURCHILL LIVINGSTONE
Medical Division of Longman Group Limited

Distributed in the United States of America by Churchill Livingstone Inc., 1560 Broadway, New York, N.Y. 10036 and by associated companies, branches and representatives throughout the world.

First edition 1979
Second edition 1984

ISBN 0 443 03000 6

British Library Cataloguing in Publication Data
Bond, Michael R.
Pain. – 2nd ed.
1. Pain
I. Title
616′.0472 RB127

Library of Congress Cataloging in Publication Data
Bond, Michael R.
Pain, its nature, analysis, and treatment.
Bibliography: p.
Includes index.
1. Pain. I. Title. [DNLM: 1. Pain WL 704 B711p]
RB127.B66 1984 616′.0472 83-7254

Printed in Singapore by Kyodo Shing Loong Printing Industries Pte Ltd

Foreword

This book deals with one of the most important concerns of humankind and one of the foremost factors that has influenced the course of history. As the records of every race and every civilization are examined, one finds ubiquitous testimonials to the omnipresence of pain. While acute pain usually serves the useful purpose of warning the individual of something wrong and prompts him or her to seek medical counsel, in many instances it is deleterious to the organism. If not promptly eliminated, postoperative pain and posttraumatic pain, and the pain of myocardial infarction and the associated reflex responses often aggravate the physiopathology and produce serious dysfunction of respiration, circulation, and other body functions. Moreover, when pain persists and becomes chronic, it imposes severe emotional, physical, economic and sociologic stresses on the patient, the family and society. As Milton so elegantly stated in *Paradise Lost* (Book 6):

> But pain is perfect miseries, the worst
> Of all evils an excessive
> Overturns all patience.

Because chronic pain is the most frequent cause of disability, it constitutes a major national and world health and economic problem. Although accurate statistics are not available, data from a variety of sources suggest that chronic pain states cost billions of pounds annually for health care services and loss of work productivity. Even more important is the cost in terms of human suffering. It is a very distressing fact that in this age of marvelous scientific and technologic advances there are millions of suffering patients who are not getting the relief they deserve. Many of these patients are exposed to high risk of iatrogenic complications from improper therapy including narcotic addiction, or subjected to multiple, often useless and, at times, mutilating operations; a significant number give up medical care and some, with severe intractable pain, become so desperate as to commit suicide.

One of the main reasons for the inadequate care of patients with pain is the void in our knowledge about basic pain mechanisms. Although much new information has been acquired during the past half century since the scientific study of pain began, much of this has not been as beneficial to patients as one might anticipate or as many people believe. This less-than-optimal payoff from the many past research efforts is due to the fact that until a decade or so ago most basic scientists working in the isolation of the animal laboratory were not concerned with ill people in pain. Moreover, the predominant concern with anatomic and physiologic research on pain consequent to the widespread assumption that pain was a purely sensory experience caused emotional and psychologic factors to be relegated secondary roles and thus discouraged psychologic research.

The second important reason for the deficiencies in managing chronic pain has been the improper or inadequate application of available knowledge. This, in turn, has been due to lack of organized teaching of medical students and physicians and other health professionals in the *proper* management of patients with pain. Consequently, many physicians do not fully appreciate the complex nature of pain and the important role that psychologic and related factors play in the pain experience. Moreover, most physicians have not been taught the indication, advantages, limitations and complications of the various modalities that are currently available for the treatment of pain.

Fortunately, during the past decade or so, several developments have taken place, which if sustained and enhanced, have the promise of increasing the capability of health professionals to cope better with this serious health problem. For one thing, there has been an impressive surge of interest among some biomedical scientists to collaborate with clinicians in studying the mechanisms and physiopathology of clinical pain syndromes. For another, a number of clinical investigators have defined more precisely the characteristics of pain and various chronic pain states. Another important series of contributions has been made by a small group of psychiatrists and psychologists whose studies have helped to define and emphasize the importance of learning and personality, and of perceptual, cultural and emotional factors on the individual's total pain experience.

Professor Bond has been at the forefront of this encouraging trend and has done an impressive series of clinical studies in patients with chronic pain. Through these studies, he has helped to clarify the role of psychologic, sociologic, and environmental factors in influencing the patient's pain behaviour and to clarify the importance of the psychodynamics of anxiety, depression, and other emotional and affective consequences of chronic pain. He has been one of the relatively few clinical investigators who have studied the psychologic and sociologic aspects of cancer pain. The publication of many of his original articles has had a very important impact on our understanding of chronic pain syndromes and consequently on improving their management.

This book represents the culmination of Professor Bond's efforts to make available information which will help physicians provide optimal care to patients with pain. The book contains a comprehensive overview of current knowledge about the neurophysiologic, psychologic and biochemical bases for pain, the clinical characteristics of pain syndromes in various body regions, and the most common therapeutic modalities in current use. The responsibility of the writer of a book of this nature is to evaluate, distill and interpret the vast amount of available information, and present it clearly and concisely. Professor Bond has met this challenge in a superb fashion. In reading the volume, one is most impressed by the distillation of the vast amount of information into such a reasonably sized book and he has discussed various aspects of pain thoroughly, lucidly and concisely. To those who know Professor Bond, the book reflects not only his intense interest in the field, but his critical analysis based on an impressive experience as a clinician and investigator and his talent and skill to communicate.

The book should prove extremely useful to medical students and students of other health professions. For this reason, the volume should be popular among medical educators who heretofore have not had a reasonably sized textbook for teaching students and physicians. For the practicing physician, the book should prove a highly effective source for the better understanding and treatment of pain. The ultimate benefit will be improved patient care which is, after all the *raison d'être* of the clinician.

Seattle, 1984

Preface to the second edition

The first edition of this book was very well received and it has been a pleasure to revise it using the helpful criticism offered by friends, other readers and by reviewers. Interest in pain and its control in those who suffer it has expanded rapidly since 1978 and this edition contains information about both the scientific discoveries of the past 6 years and recent improvements in methods of diagnosis and management. All illustrations have been redrawn and their quality has been improved considerably.

Information about advances in the understanding of the complexities of anatomical, neurophysiological and biochemical mechanisms involved in pain generation and modulation are incorporated in the first part of the book. New sections dealing with the discovery and possible functions of the opioid peptides, substance P and serotonin, have been added to Chapter 1. Fresh knowledge concerning the anatomical and physiological complexities of the 'gate mechanism' proposed by Melzack and Wall in 1965 has been summarised and incorporated in the text. Chapter 2 has been modified and expanded to include a section dealing with the prostaglandins and other chemical factors which play an important role in the first stages of pain generation.

The second, clinical part, has been revised and new sections dealing with common clinical disorders which give rise to pain in the perineum, rectum and female pelvis, have been added. Also an important section which gives details of pain terms recommended for use world-wide by The International Association for the Study of Pain has been included.

The third part of the book dealing with pain management has been revised extensively, especially Chapter 17 which deals with drugs for pain relief. A section concerning the use of biofeedback has been added to Chapter 18. Detailed tables giving guidelines to those who have to select analgesics for patients suffering acute pain following surgery or the chronic pain of malignant disease have been added to Chapters 19 and 20 respectively, thus strengthening the practical value of the book.

Finally, with the rapid expansion in knowledge there has been an accompanying increase in the number of books and articles dealing with various aspects of pain and its management. Therefore the bibliography has been revised to give the reader an opportunity to consult recently published texts which amplify ideas and techniques described briefly in this book.

Hope of improved relief for pain sufferers lies in a combination of technical developments in treatment methods based upon improved knowledge of the fundamental biological, psychological and social processes involved in pain generation and modulation, and, just as much, in continued education of all involved in patient care. This book was first written, and has now been revised, to aid the latter process and I hope that its purpose will be achieved.

1984 M.R.B.

Preface to the first edition

'For the happiness mankind can gain
Is not in pleasure, but in rest from pain'.
John Dryden (1631–1700)

This book has been written primarily for medical undergraduates in the clinical years of their studies when they have both a knowledge of basic sciences and some experience of working with patients. It is a broad-based account of the nature of pain, its meaning and significance as a symptom of physical and mental illness, and the various types of treatment available for those who suffer it. This approach is in keeping with my own belief that pain is all too often regarded merely as a symptom of physical disease or injury with scant attention to the fact that it is a personal or 'private' experience and one which varies greatly in intensity for any given disorder, both between individuals and within the same person from time to time. There are several reasons for these differences some of which are personal, others being determined by the circumstances in which pain develops; in other words, pain is a subjective experience determined by the complex interplay of biological, psychological and social factors.

In addition to understanding the nature of anatomical structures and physiological mechanisms involved in the generation of pain and modulation of its intensity, it is equally important for us to be able to recognise the different patterns of behaviour shown by people as part of the experience of being in pain. For example, the behaviour of those with similar painful disorders often differs considerably because of variations in their personality characteristics and ways of handling the stresses imposed by illness. The different patterns of behaviour are easily recognisable and should always be considered in the diagnosis and management of painful conditions. Over and above the influence of personality, the effects of the type of pain, that is whether it is acute or chronic, whether it is associated with a threat to life or not and whether it can be seen as a useful indicator of disease or as a useless and seemingly unavoidable stress as in certain chronic illnesses, also produces profoundly different patterns of behaviour. To complicate matters further, these factors must be interpreted with the sufferer's cultural and social background in mind. Finally, it is often not appreciated that complaints of pain may be quite genuine in the absence of detectable physical damage to body tissues and be a leading symptom of a disorder of emotional life, or a manifestation of abnormalities in personality development and methods of coping with life's stresses.

The issues mentioned are dealt with in the first two sections of the book entitled 'The Nature of Pain' and 'Clinical Analysis of Pain'. It will have become clear already that treatment of pain, dealt with in the final section, must be tailored to an individual's needs by taking into account physical, psychological and social factors – a process which may be quite simple, or very complex and time-consuming. There is a wide range of treatments available for pain and although a doctor cannot be skilful in all of them he or she must know the general principles of the more specialised ones in order to be able to refer patients to those trained to administer them. With this in mind all the major forms of treatment available have been described with most attention being given to those which are often used by doctors in practice in hospitals or the community.

It is hoped that this book will stimulate interest in the treatment of those in pain, and in some small way help to reduce their suffering.

1978 M.R.B.

Acknowledgements

I wish to acknowledge the helpful criticisms made by many friends and readers of the first edition of this book. Published criticisms have also been of value and the second edition incorporates many changes which will, I hope, deal with the various suggestions that have been made.

I am grateful to Mr Ian Ramsden, Head of the Medical Illustration Department in the University of Glasgow, for the considerable improvements he has made to the illustrations. Also to Mr Gordon Waddell for advice and to Drs Ian Clarke and Keith Budd for permission to use their published table of analgesics for post-operative pain.

Grateful acknowledgement is made to the following authors and publishers for permission to reproduce illustrative material from their works:

A. L. Hodgkin and The Liverpool University Press, publishers, for permission to reproduce Figure 12 from *The Conduction of The Nervous Impulse* (1964), and to W. B. Jennett and William Heinemann Medical Books Ltd., publishers, to reproduce Figure 58 from *An Introduction to Neurosurgery* (1964, first edition); R. A. Sternbach and The Academic Press Inc., publishers, to reproduce Figure 3 from Chapter 3 of *Pain Patients; Traits and Treatments* (1974), and to J. D. Morrison, W. B. Loan, J. W. Dundee and *The British Medical Journal* for permission to reproduce Tables 4 and 5 from their article 'Controlled comparison of the efficacy of fourteen preparations in the relief of post-operative pain', published in Volume 3 of *The British Medical Journal* in 1971.

My secretary, Miss B. M. Shaw has, as before, given invaluable assistance in preparing the manuscript for which I am very grateful.

Contents

PART ONE

The nature of pain

1

An anatomical basis for pain

Pain is a subjective experience arising from activity within the brain in response to damage to body tissues, to changes in the function of the brain itself either as a result of damage due to injury or disease, or to changes of a more subtle nature perhaps depending upon biochemical changes which also appear to play a role in producing mental illness. Our knowledge of the anatomical structures in the brain, the pathways along which nerve impulses giving rise to pain travel, and the biochemical mechanisms mentioned is incomplete, but in order to familiarise the reader with current views on these topics what is known of them is dealt with in outline, the first step being devoted to the understanding of the structure of nerve cells and the way in which their activity is generated and conducted through the nervous system. After that physiological and biochemical aspects of pain generation and modulation are described.

THE NEURON

The neuron, or nerve cell, consists of a cell body and two sets of processes responsible for the conduction of impulses (Fig. 1). Dendrites are short branched processes arising from the cell body. There are many of them and they increase the area of the neuron available for contact with nearby nerve cells, their dendrites and axons. The axon of a nerve is a single filament, often of considerable length, along which information is conducted from one part of the nervous system to another. Peripheral nerves consist of large numbers of axons and the major conducting pathways in the spinal cord, medulla, pons, mid-brain and sub-cortical regions are composed of them too. Their numbers are enormous and it has been estimated that in the dorsal roots of the spinal cord alone there are over a million axons, and in the brain somewhere in the order of ten billion.

Axons have a central core of axoplasm which is a viscous substance contained within a semipermiable and electrically excitable membrane. Almost all axons are invested in a spiral sheath composed of

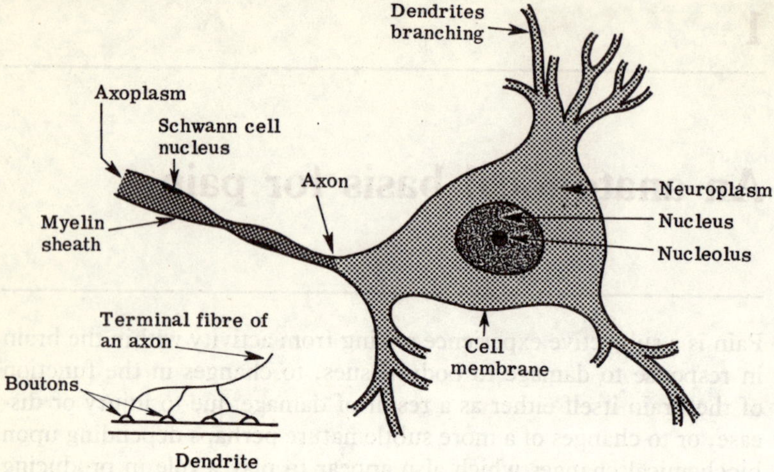

Fig 1. A neuron and it processes

a series of highly specialised cells; the Schwann cells in peripheral nerves and the oligodendrocytes in the central nervous system. These contain a lipid substance, myelin, which is an electrical insulator with a significant effect upon electrical conduction (Fig. 2). Schwann cells are similar in size and thickness and are arranged alongside each other but between them is a small bare area of axon termed a node of Renvier. Myelin influences the rate at which electrical impulses can be conducted. It is highest where the myelin is thickest and lowest where it is thinnest and it is known that neuronal conduction velocity is proportional to the square root of the diameter of the axon. The velocity at which impulses travel can be calculated on the basis of 6 metres per second per micron thickness and as neurons vary in diameter from 2 to 20 microns conduction speeds range from 12 to 120 metres per second. Some neurons have a very thin myelin sheath and, being of a diameter of 0.2 to 1 microns with insulation, their conduction rates are in the order of 0.7 to 2 metres

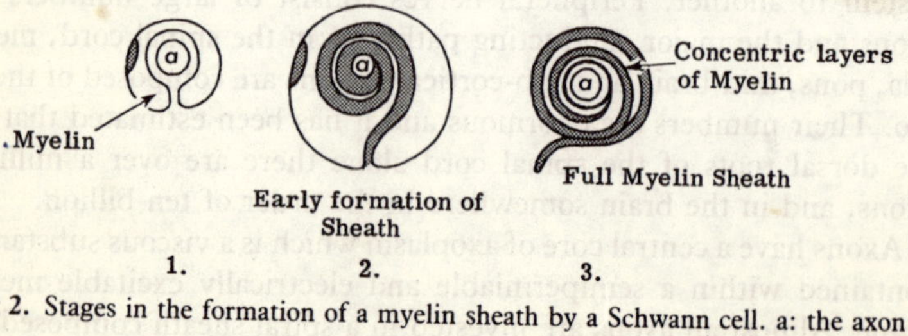

Fig 2. Stages in the formation of a myelin sheath by a Schwann cell. a: the axon

per second. Neurons of this size play a significant role in the conduction of impulses which give rise to 'slow pain' and are known as C fibres. Slightly larger fibres with a diameter of 1 to 6 microns, known as A delta fibres, conduct impulses concerned with 'fast pain' generation and they are the only ones known to be solely involved this event being activated by an intense stimulus which injures the skin, such as a pinprick.

A knowledge of the way in which nerves conduct information to the brain, or from it, is necessary for the understanding of mechanisms responsible for the generation of pain and various forms of treatment for pain relief.

THE NERVE IMPULSE

The basis of neuronal conduction is electrochemical and depends on the passage of sodium, potassium and chloride ions, to and fro across the semipermeable membrane which surrounds the central core of axoplasm. Where an axon is electrically inactive the concentration of potassium ions is greater within than without, and the reverse is true for sodium and chloride ions. The difference in concentration depends upon three factors: first the diffusion of ions (potassium and chloride moving more readily than sodium); a metabolic process known as the sodium pump which actively transports sodium ions from within the axon; and, lastly, active transfer of potassium ions into the axoplasm. The arrangement of ions in this way gives the axon a resting potential with a voltage difference across the membrane where the interior of the axon is 70 millivolts negative with respect to the exterior. When chemical or electrical stimulation of sufficient strength to alter the permeability of the semipermeable membrane occurs the distribution of ions changes. The interior of the axon becomes positively charged with respect to the exterior in the order of 40 to 50 millivolts for a brief period as sodium ions and chloride ions flow rapidly into the axon. Very shortly afterwards potassium ions flow out. This change in the electrical state is known as depolarisation and leads to sequential changes of a similar kind along the length of the axon (Figs. 3a and 3b). This results in a wave of change in the electrical state, which is the conduction of an impulse (Fig. 4). Depolarisation will not occur if the stimulus is too weak, therefore the axon gives an 'all or none' response. Electrical activity ceases for a brief period when the influx of sodium ions ceases and the membrane becomes impermeable to them; the axon is then in a refractory state. Once permeability is restored the whole process is reversed with sodium and chloride ions being pumped out

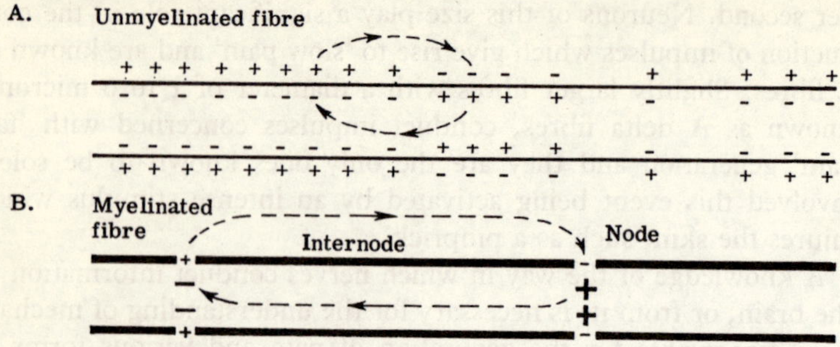

Fig 3. Propagation of impulse activity along a nerve fibre (Modified from Hodgkin 1964) A: an unmyelinated axon. B: a myelinated axon

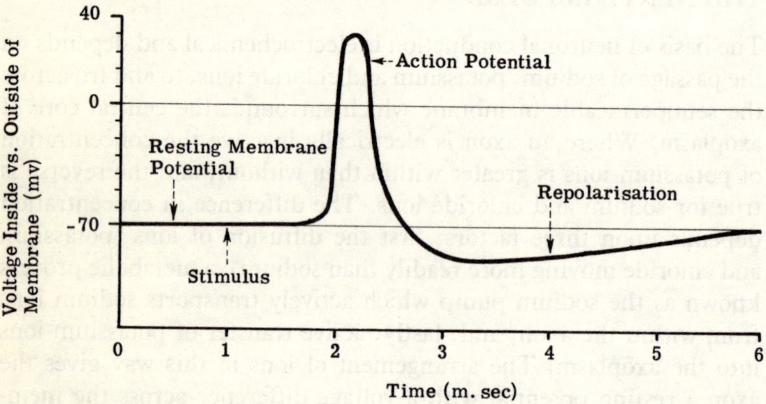

Fig 4. Electrical changes in a nerve fibre during the generation and passage of an action potential

and potassium moved into the axon to restore the negative potential, which is a process known as repolarisation. Because the axon and its immediate environment contain ions greatly in excess of the numbers required for the passage of a single impulse immediate restoration of ion balance is not necessary for the passage of further impulses and, indeed, it is only after the passage of many impulses that an axon reaches a state where conduction ceases. This will ultimately happen if stimulation is continued long enough because, although the sodium pump is in constant operation, the speed with which it effects ion transfer does not match the rate at which ion exchanges occur as the result of depolarisation.

Depolarisation causes changes in the permeability of an adjacent section of nerve preparing it for an action potential. In effect the action potential proceeds along the nerve in a continuous fashion but only if the latter does not have have a myelin sheath, namely only in the case of the smallest fibres. The presence of Schwann cells alters the method of conduction and the rate of transfer of the impulse. Electrical activity can occur only at nodal areas where the axon is not invested by myelin and. therefore, depolarisation jumps from node to node in a process called saltatory conduction (*saltare*, Latin 'to leap'). The differences in the process of electrical conduction by a myelinated and non-myelinated axon are shown in (Figs 3a and 3b).

THE SYNAPSE

Electrical activity cannot be transferred directly from one nerve to another and requires the presence of a chemical substance which is released by the process of depolarisation at the terminal of the active nerve. This is known as a transmitter substance, or neurotransmitter, and after release it travels across a narrow space to a receptor site on the body or a dendrite of the nerve to which the transfer is being made where depolarisation takes place initiating activity in the next neuron of the chain. The terminals of the transmitting nerve are known as boutons and each nerve has many of them, ending on several nerve cells and their process nearby. There are many different transmitter substances in different parts of the central nervous system and they include acetylcholine, noradrenaline, dopamine, serotonin, substance P, and the recently discovered enkephalins, met-enkephalin and leu-enkephalin. The space across which the neurotransmitter passes is the synapse and it is bounded by the membranes of the two nerves involved. In the case of the transmitting nerve this is known as the presynaptic membrane, and in the case of the receptor as the post-synaptic membrane (Fig. 5).

Electrochemical activity at a synapse depends upon the nature of the transmitter substance released and its effect upon the receptor, which varies in different parts of the nervous system. In simple terms there are two forms of synapse, the excitatory synapse, where the action potential from one nerve generates similar activity in its neighbour by causing depolarisation, and the inhibitory synapse, where the effect of the transmitter substance is to cause hyperpolarisation and resistance to the generation of an action potential in neighbouring nerve cell (Fig. 5).

Inhibition of electrical activity may occur one stage earlier at a presynaptic level where a process from a third neuron forms a second synapse on the potentially transmitting nerve. Impulses delivered by the former depolarise the pre-synaptic region of the latter causing

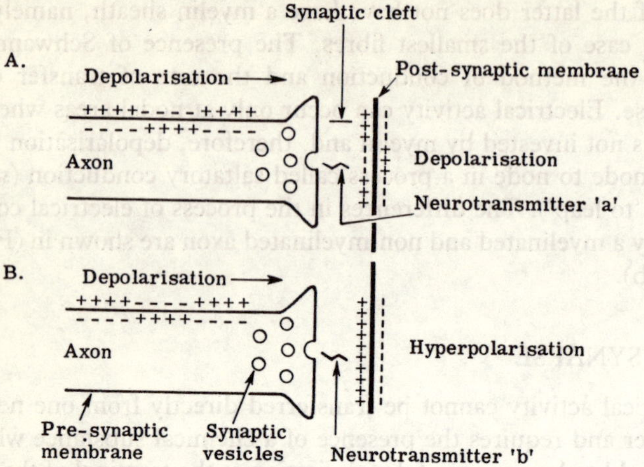

Fig 5. Conduction of nerve impulse activity at the synapse. A: an excitatory synapse B: an inhibitory synapse

a reduction in action potentials on it and consequently a reduction in the amount of transmitter substance it produces. Nerve processes which have this effect may arise from afferent nerves travelling towards the central nervous system, or from efferent nerves which have their sites of origin at a higher level. By contrast, the process of conduction across the synapse may be facilitated by the action of other nerve processes which increase the amount of neurotransmitter substance released by the transmitting nerve. Finally, inhibition may also take place at the post-synaptic membrane. This complex system of inhibitory and excitatory activity must be involved in pain modulation and, even at this stage, it becomes clear that the type of activity occuring at synapses is very important to our understanding of pain.

TRANSMISSION PATHWAYS TO THE BRAIN

Information generated by noxious stimuli reaches the brain by passage along the peripheral nerves, ascent of the spinal cord along one of a number of pathways which later traverse the medulla and mid-brain terminating in the thalamus, from where distribution to the cerebral cortex occurs. Peripheral neurons, in which the original stimulus generates information, synapse in the region of the dorsal horns of the spinal cord, and these are called the first order neurons. Second order neurons either travel the length of the cord to reach the thalamus, or are represented by a series of short interconnected neurons which eventually reach centres in the medulla, midbrain and thalamus. The former acts as a fast conducting pathway for pricking or sharp pain and the latter as a slow conducting pathway for dull, diffuse and more persistent pain.

PERIPHERAL NERVE

Following noxious stimulation volleys of impulses pass along nerve fibres in the sensory component of mixed peripheral nerves entering the spinal cord through its dorsal roots where the cell bodies of the nerves lie within the dorsal root ganglion. The fibres traverse the lateral aspect of the dorsal root and their sites of termination include the tract of Lissauer and sites in the dorsal horns of the grey matter of the spinal cord (Fig. 6). Recently anatomists have demonstrated that approximately one-third of all afferent small diameter C fibres enter the spinal cord through its anterior roots and travel to the dorsal horns to join C fibres which entered via the posterior roots. Their cell bodies are also within the dorsal root ganglia.

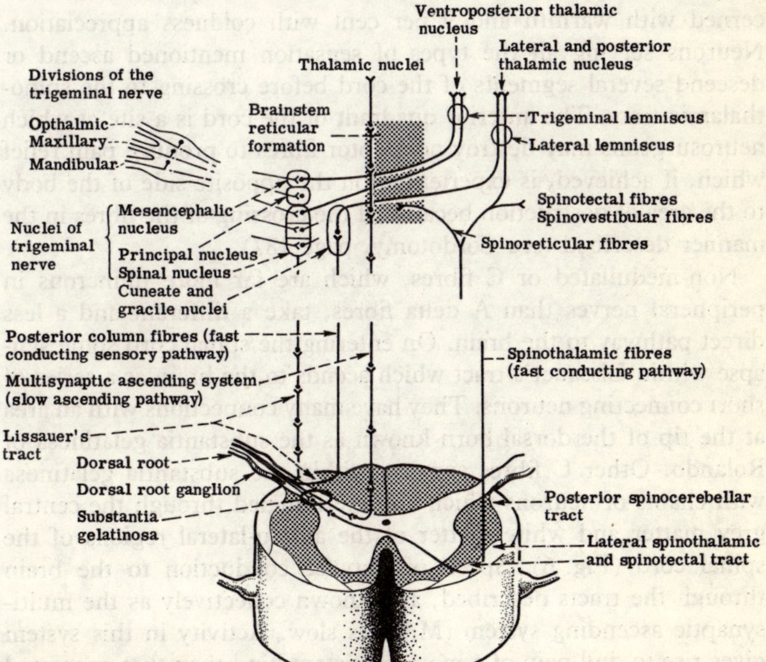

Fig 6. Pathways in the spinal cord and brain for the conduction of 'fast' and 'slow' pain

SPINAL CORD PATHWAYS

Neurons of the A delta group are responsible for rapid transmission of impulses to the brain ultimately giving rise to the 'sharp' or 'bright' elements of 'fast pain'. This is best illustrated by considering the effects of a burn which produces a rapid withdrawal from the stimulus with an accompanying sharp pain followed by dull pain of long duration. Incoming A delta neurons, synapse in the nucleus proprius of the dorsal horn of the spinal cord, and their second order neurons then cross in front of the central canal to reach the lateral spinothalamic tract in which they ascend ultimately reaching the thalamus (Fig. 6). Thus there is only one synapse in this pathway between the peripheral stimulus and the brain. The spinothalamic tract, often represented as having an anterior and lateral component, also carries neurons, the activity of which ultimately gives rise to the sensations of warmth and coldness and which have crossed the cord following the same route as nociceptor fibres (pain fibres). It has been estimated that in the spinothalamic tracts about 54 per cent of neurons are concerned with pain generation and 46 per cent with temperature appreciation. Of the latter about 37 per cent are concerned with warmth and 9 per cent with coldness appreciation. Neurons serving all the types of sensation mentioned ascend or descend several segments of the cord before crossing to the spinothalamic tract. The anterior quadrant of the cord is a site at which neurosurgeons may destroy nociceptor fibres to produce pain relief which, if achieved, is experienced on the opposite side of the body to the area of destruction because of the crossing of the fibres in the manner described (see Cordotomy, page 187).

Non-medullated or C fibres, which are far more numerous in peripheral nerves than A delta fibres, take a different and a less direct pathway to the brain. On entering the spinal cord some synapse within Lissauer's tract which acends to the brain as a series of short connecting neurons. They have many connections with an area at the tip of the dorsal horn known as the substantia gelatinosa of Rolando. Other C fibres synapse within the substantia gelatinosa with chains of neurons which are intermingled through the central grey matter and white matter of the antero-lateral regions of the spinal cord (Fig. 6). Speed of impulse conduction to the brain through the tracts described, and known collectively as the multisynaptic ascending system (MAS) is slow. Activity in this system gives rise to dull pain of a more persistent kind than that generated by activity in the spinothalamic tract. Neurons in Lissauer's tract and the substantia gelatinosa join the spinal nucleus of the trigeminal nerve (the fifth cranial nerve) which receives nociceptor fibres from the head. From this point further neurons carry information either across the midline to nuclei in the thalamus, or into the central grey matter where they enter the brain stem reticular formation which has rich connections with the thalamus, hypothalamus, basal ganglia and cerebral cortex. 'Pain' afferent fibres also travel in the glosso-pharyngeal nerve (the ninth cranial nerve) and the vagus nerve (the tenth cranial nerve) from the structures in the ear, pharynx and larynx.

PATHWAYS IN THE MEDULLA AND MID-BRAIN

The fast conducting neurons of the spinothalamic tracts, accompanied by other sensory neurons and those from the sensory nucleus of the trigeminal nerve in which neurons giving rise to sharp pain from the head travel, pass towards the thalamus as part of the lateral lemniscus and trigeminal lemniscus, their final destination being the ventrobasal nuclear complex of that structure (Fig. 7). During their passage many neurons from the tracts turn into the brain stem reticular formation about which the remainder appear to form a par-

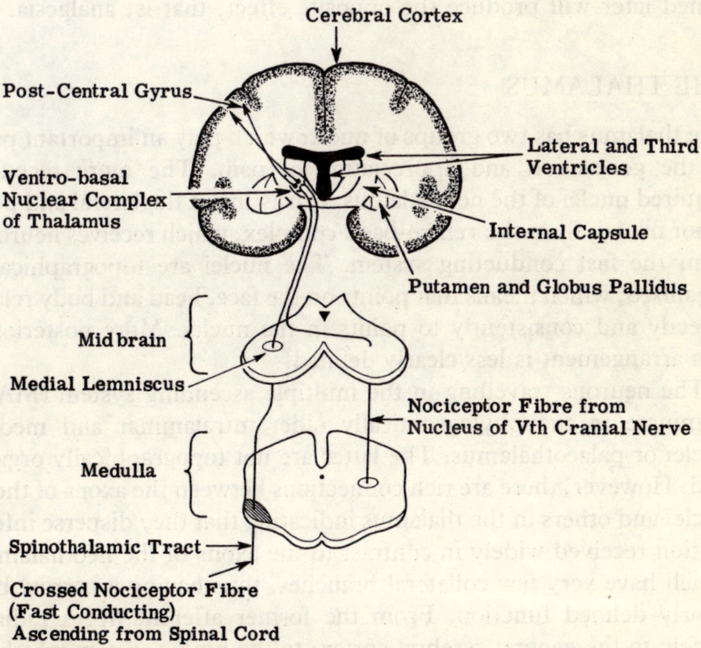

Fig 7. Conduction pathways for facial, trunk and limb pain

tial sheath. Stimulation of this outer zone of the brain stem in man gives rise to bright, sharp or burning pain, and also a sensation of coldness. The experience is felt over the opposite side of the face and body and is accompanied by autonomic changes too, namely the erection of hairs and sweating.

The fibres of the multisynaptic ascending system (MAS), including those from the lowermost parts of the spinal nucleus of the trigeminal nerve, synapse with the cells of brain stem reticular formation which forms a central core of diffusely arranged grey matter. Fibres from the reticular formation radiate to all areas of the cortex, thereby alerting it to the effects of sensory stimuli of all kinds. Information arising as a result of peripheral noxious stimulation and activation of sufficient numbers of cells in the reticular formation passes from the latter to both the intralaminar and medial nuclei of the thalamus, to the hypothalamus, and other areas of the brain concerned with autonomic activities and emotion. Stimulation of the central grey matter of the brain stem in a conscious patient will, in certain areas, produce a diffuse burning or cold sensation in the head and trunk, intense dread and fear, and autonomic changes including erection of hair and increase in heart rate and sweating on the opposite side of the body. Stimulation in other areas to be mentioned later will produce the opposite effect, that is, analgesia.

THE THALAMUS

The thalamus has two groups of nuclei which play an important part in the generation and appreciation of pain. The more recently acquired nuclei of the neothalamus, consisting of the lateral and posterior nuclei, form the ventro-basal complex, which receives neurons from the fast conducting system. The nuclei are topographically organised, which means that points on the face, head and body relate directly and consistently to points in the nuclei. More posteriorly this arrangement is less clearly defined.

The neurons travelling in the multiple ascending system (MAS) terminate in the phylogenetically older intralaminar and medial nuclei or palaeothalamus. The latter are not topographically organised. However, there are rich connections between the axons of these nuclei and others in the thalamus indicating that they disperse information received widely in contrast to the axons of the neothalamus which have very few collateral branches, thus having a narrow but clearly defined function. From the former afferent fibres radiate widely to the general cerebral cortex, to the limbic system which is concerned with emotion and memory, and to the basal ganglia which are concerned with movement control. They do not send afferent fibres to the primary sensory areas of the cortex, but on the other hand fibres from the neothalamus only radiate to this area of the brain where there is a topographical arrangement reflecting that in the thalamus.

THE CEREBRAL CORTEX

Although direct electrical stimulation of the cerebral cortex does not give rise to pain in a conscious individual, whereas thalamic stimulation will do so, the different regions of the cortex are essential if the site of stimulation or damage is to be accurately located, if the quality of the stimulus is to be judged, if it is to be compared with past experience, and if it is to take on its normal emotional qualities.

Sensory discrimination involves registration of information about a noxious stimulus leading to its location on or within the body through the generation of proprioceptive activity and sensations, such as touch, warmth, pressure and, furthermore, it also includes the assessment of the magnitude of the stimulus. This activity is aroused by transmission through the lateral spinothalamic tract, and posterior column fibres which terminate in the somatosensory cortex of the post-central gyrus, the posterior paracentral gyrus, and the cortex of the parietal operculum. Of these three areas the last two seem to be associated more closely with pain than the first. The cortex of the Island of Reil, which lies buried in the Sylvian fissure between the frontal and temporal lobes, is involved in the experience of visceral pain. Emotional aspects of pain and the responses associated with it are generated within the limbic system. This was first described by Papez in 1935 and his concepts were later extended by others, although from the late 19th century, when the eminent French neurologist, Broca, commented that the cortical area at the base of the hemispheres is the site of 'man's brute instincts', knowledge of the function of this region has been emerging. Damage to any of these areas leads to distortion of the pain experience. For example, following a modified leucotomy in which fronto-thalamic tracts involved in emotional activity are cut, patients continue to locate pain and describe its character accurately but lose the emotional experience of unpleasantness.

PATHWAYS FOR FACIAL PAIN

Stimulation of the skin of the face and structures within the mouth and nasal sinuses generates activity within fibres of one of the three divisions of the trigeminal nerve, which are represented in the face by its ophthalmic, maxillary and mandibular branches. Having entered the skull separately the divisions join to form the trigeminal ganglion where the cell bodies lie and from which fibres travel onwards to terminate at one of three nuclei in the brain stem (Fig. 6). Proprioceptor fibres for facial and orbital muscles, muscles of mastication and the tongue, pass to the mesencephalic nucleus, a proportion of the fibres subserving touch and pressure pass to the principle nucleus, with the remainder, together with fibres for pain and temperature joining together to form the spinal tract of the trigeminal nerve, which is a long body extending downwards through the medulla and beyond to the level of the fourth cervical segment. Fibres within the spinal tract turn medially into the spinal nucleus of the trigeminal nerve where those for pain terminate at its lower levels. The arrangement of fibres at this point is curious for it seems that those for the central part of the face terminate at a higher level than those for the most lateral parts, with the mid-zones being represented by the intermediate area of the nucleus.

A second series of neurons travels from the sensory nucleus across the midline carrying information for thermal and pricking pain receptors to the trigeminal lemniscus which lies lateral to the medial lemniscus. Information is carried to the medial part of the ventro-posterior nucleus of the thalamus where it is represented somatotopically. Information from the lowest or most caudal part of the sensory nucleus where input is from fibres representing poorly localised sensations, including pain; travels to the reticular formation for distribution to the intralaminar nucleus of the thalamus.

From the ventro-posterior nucleus of the thalamus nerve fibres for touch and pressure radiate to the post central gyrus of the sensory cortex via the posterior limb of the internal capsule reaching its lower part. Information that has reached the intralaminar nucleus of the thalamus is distributed through the diffuse thalamic projection system to the cortex. An overall diagramatic representation of the distribution of neuronal activity from the reticular formation and thalamus to the cerebral cortex is given in Figure 8.

In addition to peripheral afferents, descending neurons from higher centres also take part in the 'gate control' mechanism. It is believed that activity in enkephalinergic cells in the periaqueductal grey matter of the brain stem excites serotonergic cells in a nearby nucleus (the dorsal raphe nucleus) which, in turn, activates a third series of nerve cells in a midline structure of the lower brain stem and medulla (the nucleus raphe magnus). The axons of these serotonergic cells travel in the dorsolateral columns of the spinal cord

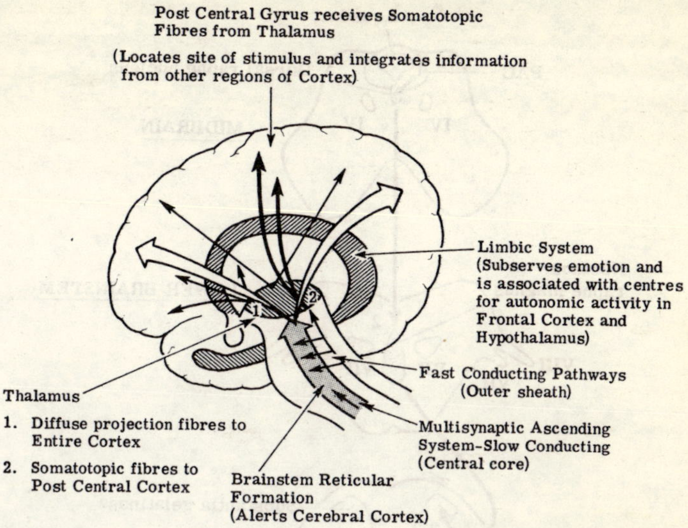

Fig 8. Functions of the cerebral cortex and reticular formation of the brain stem in pain generation

and terminate in the substantia gelatinosa of the dorsal horns where they excite small enkephalinergic interneurons as shown in Figures 9 and 14. These inhibit other cells which form part of the afferent neuronal chain.

THE AUTONOMIC NERVOUS SYSTEM AND PAIN

The autonomic nervous system controls the activities of the heart, viscera, glands, blood vessels and smooth muscle and because the activity of these organs only occasionally intrudes into consciousness and because they function without conscious control the system is also known as the involuntary or vegetative nervous system. There are two anatomically and physiologically distinct components of the autonomic nervous system which act synergistically where they innervate the same organ, for example the eye and the heart. They are known as the sympathetic and parasympathetic systems. Apart from acting synergistically they may also act alone, for example the sympathetic system supplies the uterus and renal medulla and arterioles, and the parasympathetic system the glands of the stomach and pancreas.

Afferent fibres carrying information, resulting from noxious stimulation from the periphery to the central nervous system travel from the viscera and from non-visceral structures. They are sympathetic

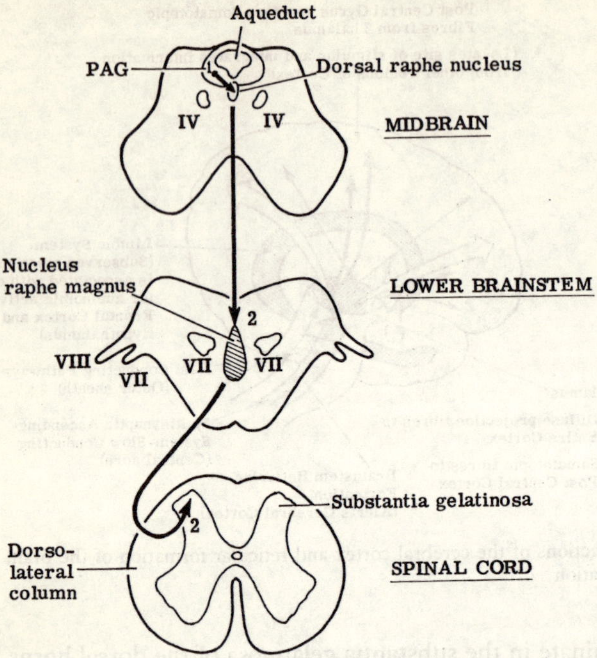

Fig 9. Inhibitory efferent pathways which influence modulation of afferent nerve impulses in the dorsal horns of the spinal cord. 1. enkephalinergic cells, 2. serotonergic cells.

nerve fibres chiefly and their cell bodies lie in the dorsal root ganglia from which central processes travel into the spinal cord where in the dorsal horn region they synapse with connector neurons (Fig. 10). Clearly, as both somatic and autonomic afferent neurons synapse in this region there is a likelihood of interaction between them and,

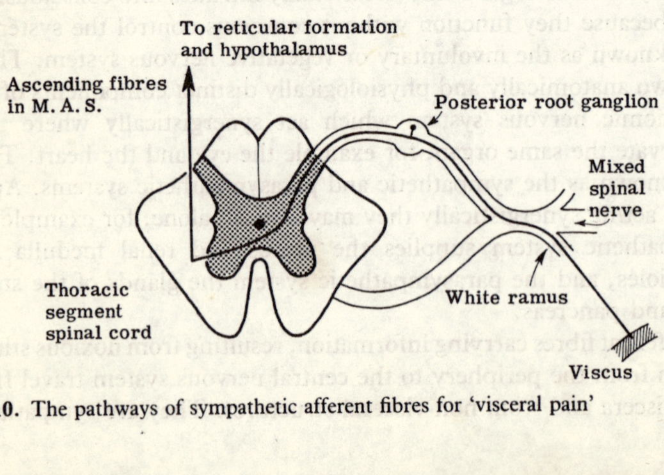

Fig 10. The pathways of sympathetic afferent fibres for 'visceral pain'

indeed, this is the case being the basis of an important phenomenon known as 'referred pain' which will be described in more detail later (see page 19).

The connector neurons either return to the periphery where they activate excitatory neurons as part of an autonomic reflex arc, or they travel to higher centres in the reticular formation of the brain stem and the hypothalamus from which high level control of autonomic function is mediated.

The pathway to the brain is probably similar to that taken by somatic afferent C fibres, namely the multiple ascending system (MAS). After synapsing in the reticular formation, which contains both sympathetic and parasympathetic areas, other neurons travel to the hypothalamus in the anterior part of which lie many centres concerned with parasympathetic activity and in the posterior part of which there are many concerned with sympathetic activity. To complete the afferent system neurons radiate from hypothalamic centres to the anterior and medial nuclei of the thalamus and then to the cerebral cortex. They also travel directly to the limbic system and thus the localisation, such as it is, the quality and significance of noxious stimuli together with their emotional loading are integrated.

Efferent connector neurons of the autonomic nervous system are present in only three regions of the nervous system:

1. In the brain in relation to the nuclei of the third, seventh, ninth and tenth cranial nerves.
2. The entire thoracic region of the spinal cord and first two lumbar segments (T1 to 12, L1 and 2).
3. The second and third sacral segments of the spinal cord.

Regions 1 and 3 form the outflow for the para-sympathetic system and region 2 for the sympathetic nervous system. Therefore they form the cranial and sacral autonomic and sympathetic systems.

The fate of the efferent connector neuron is to synapse with an excitatory neuron. This happens peripherally at sites where these cells collect to form 'ganglia' lying at some distance from the organ to be supplied in the case of the sympathetic system, or close to it, or within it in the case of the cranial and sacral autonomic systems. Bearing in mind the relationship of the connector neurons to the cell bodies of the excitatory neurons they are conventionally referred to as pre-ganglionic neurons.

The path taken by connector neurons of the sympathetic system in the thoracic region of the spinal cord is shown in Figure 11. Having left the cord in the anterior root the neuron reaches a pre-vertebral

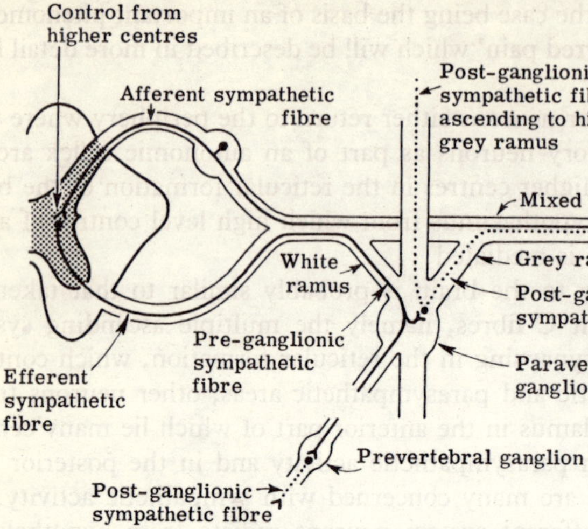

Fig 11. Pathways of sympathetic afferent and efferent fibres at spinal cord level

ganglion of the sympathetic chain via a white ramus, so called because pre-ganglionic fibres have a myelin sheath. The neuron may then:

1. Pass on to a pre-vertebral ganglion, that is the superior mesenteric, the coeliac and hypogastric ganglia.
2. Synapse with an excitatory neuron, which leaves the pre-vertebral ganglion in a grey ramus, so called because the neurons in it do not have myelin sheaths, to join a mixed peripheral nerve for distribution to blood vessels, sweat glands and the erector muscles of hairs. They are referred to as post-ganglionic neurons. They may leave to enter a mixed peripheral nerve at the same level, or travel in the sympathetic chain some distance before doing so. In the cervical region of the spinal cord there are only grey rami because pre-ganglionic sympathetic outflow takes place between the first thoracic and second lumbar segments of the spinal cord.

The fact that autonomic and somatic sensory neurons travel together in peripheral nerves is of significance in understanding the development of the condition known as causalgia after nerve damage. Sometimes injury is followed by the development of a persistent and very unpleasant burning pain (p. 120), the origin of which appears to be some form of interaction between sympathetic and damaged somatic afferent neurons. This is associated with a persistent alteration in activity in the dorsal horn region of the spinal cord and, as a consequence, the generation of constant pain which may be relieved by a sympathectomy.

The neurotransmitter in the peripheral autonomic system for all ganglia is acetylcholine. The neurotransmitter produced by excitatory neurons in the sympathetic system is noradrenaline, except in the case of sweat glands where it is acetylcholine. The neurotransmitter produced by parasympathetic excitatory neurons is acetylcholine.

Because the sensory innervation of the viscera is sparse we have a poorly developed image of our internal organs with the result that when pain is experienced it is poorly localised and dull, lacking the sharpness of pain from better innervated regions. This is not an entirely true statement because the pain of distension of the gut, known as colic, and the pain from myocardial infarction, have a very distinct quality which enables the clinician to locate the source of it with some accuracy. In the case of viscera, stimuli which give rise to pain are either chemical, such as the products of inflammation or gastric contents spilled into the peritoneum after perforation of the stomach or duodenum, or distension. They are virtually insensitive to cutting, burning and crushing. Referred pain is a further type of pain which has a considerable value in clinical practice and arises as the result of noxious stimulation of the viscera and nearby structures, such as the pleura or peritoneum, which are more richly innervated.

REFERRED PAIN

Pain arising from structures deep in the body, for example gallbladder or heart, occurs both at the site of the organ concerned and also at others more distant. For example, inflammation of the gallbladder gives rise to pain in the region of the tip of the right shoulder because the nerve roots supplying it and the adjacent diaphragmatic peritoneum are the third, fourth and fifth cervical, and the sensory dermatome at the point of the shoulder is the fifth cervical. The phenomenon described is so consistent throughout mankind as to be of considerable value in clinical diagnosis and the reason for it appears to lie in the convergence and summation of somatic and autonomic nerve impulses in the grey matter of the dorsal horns of the spinal cord. Here the effect of summation of activity and its spread is to lower the threshold for transmission of information from the skin and the sufferer gives preferential attention to it because cutaneous innervation is more strongly represented at the cerebral level. The skin of an area to which pain is referred becomes hypersensitive, and within it are small regions, known as trigger areas, which, if subjected to pressure give rise to pain both in the referred area and at the site of noxious stimulation. Anaesthesia of trigger points reduces or abolishes pain by lowering the afferent barrage from the skin, thereby lowering the amount of information reaching the dorsal horns to a level below which transmission occurs.

2

Physiological and biochemical mechanisms of pain modulation

RECEPTIVE MECHANISMS AND PATTERNS OF NERVE IMPULSE TRANSMISSION

The means by which noxious stimuli eventually give rise to pain has been a subject of discussion for centuries. Stimuli, such as heat, cold, touch and pressure, however produced, always give rise to the same sensation and it is well known that if the same stimuli are increased above a certain threshold pain occurs. These observations led to two of the early theories about the generation of pain. The first suggests that each sensation has its own receptors which respond only to a particular stimulus (Fig. 12). Support for this idea reached its peak in the second half of the 19th century when pain was regarded as a sensory experience rather like heat and cold. In 1894 Von Frey stated that each sensory modality had a specific receptor, basing his views on work indicating that the skin contains very small highly specialised areas responding to particular stimulus types such as heat or cold but to no other. The hypothesis received further support from those who identified the so called 'end organs' which were named after them, including the cold bulb of Krause, the heat organs of Ruffini and Meissner's corpuscles for touch. It was thought that pain arose by stimulation of a fine network of small nerve fibres and 'free' endings which, however, have not yet been demonstrated satisfactorily. The very high degree of specificity once described does not exist, though experimental work in animals suggests that there are cutaneous receptors which are specific for mechanical and thermal stimuli and that there are cells within the dorsal horns of the spinal cord which are activated only when the skin is warmed or cooled or when hair movement takes place. It has been demonstrated that A delta fibres are activated by high intensity stimuli and C fibres by mechanical, thermal or chemical stimuli of high intensity. In any specificity theory of pain there must be an explanation for two forms of pain experienced, as in the case of burning where there is an initially short-lived sharp or bright pain fol-

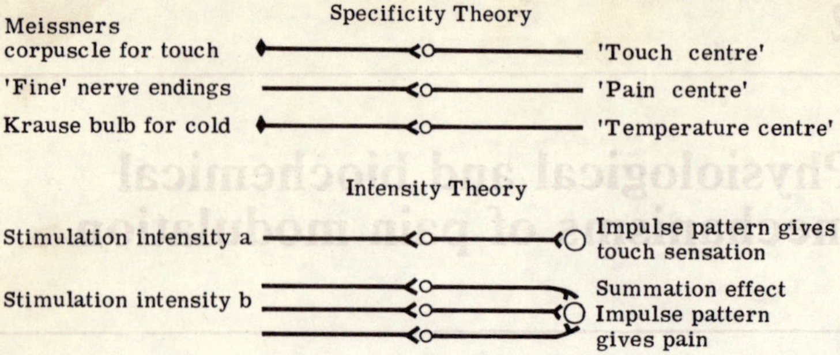

Fig 12. A diagrammatic representation of the specificity and intensity theories of pain modulation

lowed by a duller and more prolonged pain. The two forms of pain suggest the presence of specific rapid and slow conducting systems and at the present time it is generally accepted that A delta fibres are involved in the generation of sharp pain and C fibres of dull persistent pain.

A second theory of pain, which directly opposes the first, has existed for centuries and arises from the observation that a stimulus of any kind, if great enough, gives rise to pain (Fig. 12). In other words pain is merely due to the intensity of stimulation involved, the necessary condition for its arousal being the breaking of a certain threshold.

In summary, the two theories are:

1. A sensory theory which proposes that pain is a sensory phenomenon in its own right with specific receptors, routes of transmission through the central nervous system, and centres of registration, appreciation and interpretation in the brain.

2. An intensity theory which takes the view that specific receptors for pain do not exist and that pain arises as a result of stimulation by any means so long as the intensity of that stimulation passes a certain threshold.

Nowadays it is accepted that elements of both theories are necessary to a general theory of pain. For example, there are nerve fibres which are specific for pain, and again, stimulation of non-specific fibres may give rise to pain, and also to other forms of sensation too, depending upon the strength of the stimulus supplied and the pattern or coding of neural impulses that results. A modern view of the conditions in the nervous system necessary for the generation of pain incorporates the elements of both theories and has been summarised by Professor Ronald Melzack of Montreal who proposes that any theory of pain must satisfy the following criteria:

1. It must take account of the fact that the specificity of function exists in the central nervous system.
2. It must take account of the importance of temporal sequences of impulses and the summation of impulses in pain generation.
3. It must take account of the clinical observation that pain can become a persistent phenomenon in certain neurological disorders.
4. It must take account of the role played by emotion in the experience of pain and associated behaviour.

These factors were incorporated into a theory proposed by Melzack and Wall in 1965 which provided a possible explanation for the neurophysiological basis of pain modulation at the spinal cord level. The 'gate theory' provided a model which demonstrated the way in which neuronal impulses generated by noxious stimuli might be controlled in the dorsal horns of the spinal cord and their work has been the focus of considerable research in the past 17 years. There is strong evidence for a basic modulating system in the spinal cord and at higher levels too, and current views on its mode of action are discussed in the remainder of this chapter.

THE GATE THEORY

In general terms, the theory proposed by Melzack and Wall stated that information arising as a result of noxious stimulation is modified in its passage from peripheral nerve fibres to those in the spinal cord by the action of a specialised 'gating' mechanism situated in the region of the dorsal horns of the cord. Put simply, they said if the gate is in an 'open' position information is transmitted to the brain, but if partially open or closed lesser amounts of information, or none at all, reach the brain. The 'setting' of the gate and therefore the ease with which information leading to pain generation passes through it depends upon the balance of activity in large and small afferent nerve fibres, and in fibres descending from higher centres.

On the basis of experiments and deductions from histological studies, Melzack and Wall identified structures in the substantia gelatinosa and grey matter of the dorsal horns of the spinal cord which they believed formed the cellular elements of the gate system and these are illustrated diagramatically in (Fig. 13). They stated that central transmission to the brain depends upon activation of the transmission cell (T) by large or small nerve fibres. The amount of transmission from these fibres to the T cell is governed in turn by

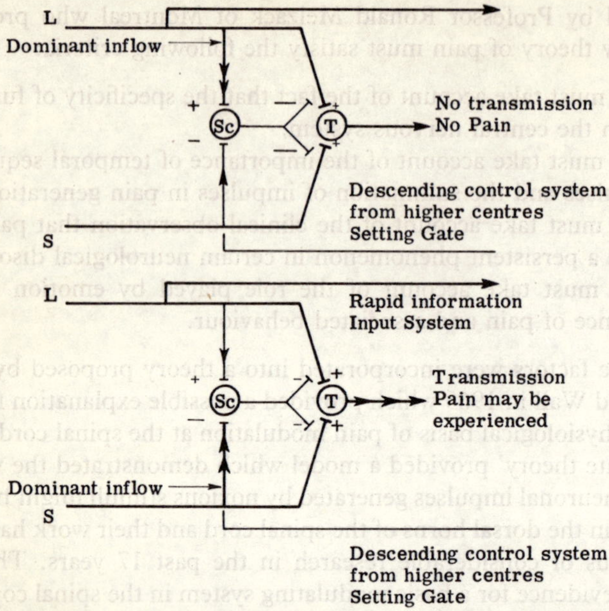

Fig 13. A diagrammatic representation of the gate theory of pain modulation

the action of a further cell in the substantia gelatinosa (the SG cell) which produces its effect by pre-synaptic and perhaps post-synaptic inhibition. The SG cell is activated by collateral branches from large fibres, chiefly those ascending in the dorsal columns of the spinal cord dealing with proprioception and touch (Aβ neurons) and it is inhibited by small fibre activity, namely those known to be concerned with pain generation. In normal circumstances the activity of the large fibre system predominates and T cell transmission is inhibited.

It was stated that in the absence of noxious stimulation there is a low but constant rate of activity in small fibres which plays a part in maintaining a state of readiness to transmit when the number of nerve impulses rises in association with noxious stimulation. When the latter occurs there is generally simultaneous activity in the large fibre system which initially inhibits discharge of the T cell by action upon the SG cell. However, summation takes place in the small fibre system and activity reaches a point at which the SG cell is inhibited by it and the T cell becomes active, the gate is opened and transmission to the brain takes place. As stated, the balance of activity in the two fibre systems is important and should the large fibre system be stimulated, as it is in everyday life when we rub an injured part of the body briskly, inhibition of further transmission takes place. Central activity also influences the situation for it may both facilitate or inhibit the passage of information centrally. Thus, in heightened anxiety the level of pain experienced is increased, because it seems that activity generated in the limbic system of the brain and transmitted via the reticular formation of the brain stem 'opens the gate'. However, in other situations, for example where an individual is engaged in a sporting contest, pain may not be experienced when an injury occurs, perhaps due to the inhibitory effect of other higher centres which 'close the gate'. So far what has been said suggests that the gate system operates only within the spinal cord but similar mechanisms are present at all levels of the central nervous system.

Experimental work has increased our understanding of the way in which modulation occurs at the spinal level. It has been confirmed that neurons involved are sited in the substantia gelatinosa of the grey matter in the dorsal horns of the spinal cord. Ideas concerning the precise mechanism of modulation have developed around the studies of both the relationship between neurons of different types, especially those influencing the function of C fibres, and upon the nature and action of the transmitter substances involved. Current theories suggest that the neurotransmitter for C fibres is substance P. Substance P is an 11-amino acid peptide first extracted from horse intestine and brain by von Euler and Gaddum in 1931. It is concentrated in several areas of the nervous system, including those known to be involved in pain generation. Laboratory experiments show:

1. Substance P is found in small neurons of sensory ganglia, in the C fibres of sensory nerves and nociceptive neurons of the trigeminal nuclei.
2. In the spinal cord, substance P is concentrated in the substantia gelatinosa which has also a high density of enkephalin-containing short interneurons. Analogues of enkephalin completely suppress the release of substance P—an action which can be reversed by the narcotic antagonist naloxone.
3. When applied to the dorsal horn of the spinal cord, substance P chiefly activates neurons which respond to noxious stimuli at the periphery.
4. The distribution of substance P in the brain is similar to that of the enkephalins.
5. The neurons of the raphe nuclei of the lower brain stem and medulla contain both substance P and serotonin which are thought

to play an important part in the modulation of pain at the spinal cord level. The excitatory effect of substance P upon the post-synaptic membrane of cells within the substantia gelatinosa is inhibited by enkephalins produced by short spinal inter-neurons which have been excited by the serotonergic neurons descending from the midline nuclei of the brain stem and medulla, (Figs 9 and 14).

6. Exogenous opiates inhibit the action of substance P and abolish pain.

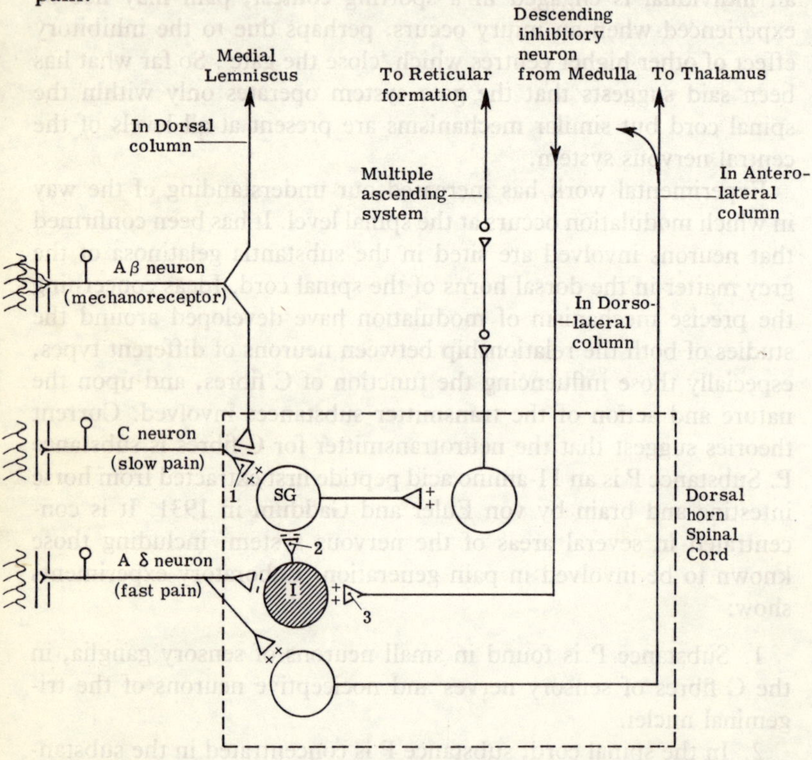

Fig 14. Modulation of afferent neurons in the dorsal horns of the spinal cord concerned with pain generation. Neurotransmitter substances: 1. substance P, 2. enkephalins, 3. serotonin. SG: substantia gelatinosa transmission cell. I: enkephalinergic inter-neuron

Figure 14 is an up-to-date simplified view of the gate mechanism incorporating the interactions of Aβ, Aδ and C afferent neurons with each other, and the putative roles of enkephalinergic inter-neurons in the substantia gelatinosa and terminals of descending serotonergic neurons in the medulla. It will be seen that the nature of the neurotransmitters at several sites is not known with certainty. It has become clear also that neurons are capable of producing more than one transmitter substance (for example, the descending serotonergic neurons also contain substance P). Thus, as in the case of the original concept put forward by Melzack and Wall, the neuro-chemical model currently under investigation represents part of the gradual unfolding of knowledge about pain modulation and it acts as a basis for further laboratory studies.

BRAIN AMINES, NARCOTIC ANALGESICS AND PAIN

Opioid peptides

In 1969 it was first shown that electrical stimulation in the periaqueductal grey matter of the brain stem of the rat causes diminution or abolition of responses to noxious stimuli. Stimulation of the same site in humans carried out much later produced similar effects and we know now that at the time of stimulation endogenous opiate substances are released. It has been known for some time that morphine acts at several sites in the brain stem and spinal cord to produce pain relief and that electrical stimulation of these sites leads to the release of endogenous opiates. Furthermore, experiments on cats show that morphine, acting at sites in the dorsal horns of the spinal cord, suppresses the activity of incoming non-myelinated C neurons and A delta neurons without affecting larger diameter fibres, (see Fig. 14). Significantly, all these effects are reversed by the morphine antagonist naloxone which also inhibits electrically induced analgesia caused by stimulation of morphine binding sites in the brain stem. The results of these experiments suggest that the nervous system contains opiate receptors, a view first substantiated by several researchers in the 1970s. The first report of the isolation of a morphine-like factor in the brain was made by Dr Hughes of Aberdeen in 1975 and this was quickly followed in the same year by the announcement by Dr Hughes, Professor Kosterlitz and others of the recovery from pig brain of two peptides with opioid activity. The substances were named enkephalins. They are pentapeptides differing only at the fifth amino acid residue and have the following general structure:

H. Tyrosine, Glycine, Phenylalanine R. OH

where R is methionine or leucine.

These substances have pharmacological properties which parallel those of morphine and related compounds, including power to produce analgesia, nausea, respiratory depression, decreased propulsion of the gut, to cause tolerance and to alter mood. Also, like morphine, their actions are opposed by the morphine antagonist naloxone.

Hughes and his co-workers observed that methionine enkephalin (met-enkephalin) had an amino acid sequence identical to the 61–65 amino acids of a pituitary hormone β-lipotropin (LPH) and it was noted that the complete terminal portion of β-LPH (amino acids 61–91) had potent opioid activity—this fragment of β-LPH is known as β-endorphin.

The opioid receptor system is far more complex than originally imagined and pain modulation is only one facet of its functions. It has been shown that β-endorphin and ACTH are present together in the pituitary gland and that they are released simultaneously in response to stress. They have a common precursor which is a very large molecule known as pro-opiocortin. Therefore, at present it is known that there are two opioid peptide systems in the brain. First the enkephalins, which are widely distributed with high concentrations in the corpus striatum, the periaqueductal grey matter of the brain stem and the dorsal horns of the spinal cord. They are also found in the cortex but in low concentrations. The enkephalins have a very short half-life and appear to be neurotransmitters concerned with pain modulation. In contrast, β-endorphin occurs in a single system which includes the anterior pituitary, medial thalamus and central brain stem. It has a much longer half-life than the enkephalins. Its function is unknown but its presence is associated with the release of prolactin, growth hormone and pitressin. As far as pain is concerned, it may well cause a more prolonged diminution of pain than the enkephalins.

A number of clinical observations support the conclusions from laboratory experiments which have demonstrated that opioid peptides are important in pain modulation. First, stimulation of periaqueductal grey matter in man leads to pain reduction and a rise in the level of opioid activity in the CSF. Second, in patients with chronic pain, levels of opioid activity in the CSF appear to be reduced and, third, patients with pain without an obvious organic cause have normal levels of opioid activity in the CSF.

Serotonin (5-Hydroxytryptamine)

Experimental observations of the effects of various drugs upon chronic pain in man have revealed that, in addition to certain opioid peptides acting as probable neurotransmitter substances, serotonin, a brain amine, is also an important neurotransmitter in systems which modulate pain. Thus it is known that:

1. Substances exist which inhibit serotonin synthesis (p-chloro-

phenylalanine), and impair electrically induced analgesia brought about by stimulation of morphine-binding sites.

2. Substances such as 5-hydroxytryptophan, a serotonin precursor, increase the level of brain serotonin and increase the level of analgesia obtained by electrical stimulation.

3. If the level of all monoamine transmitters in the brain is reduced (i.e. by tetrabenazine), or if dopamine receptor sites are blocked by drugs of the phenothiazine group (haloperidol), then analgesia cannot be obtained by electrical stimulation. Dopamine is a precursor of the neurotransmitter substance, noradrenaline.

4. If the levels of dopamine precursors are raised with levadopa, or by using a dopamine stimulating substance, such as apomorphine, analgesia is increased.

The facts mentioned illustrate that an increasingly complex system for pain modulation is being developed. It seems that electrical stimulation of selected sites in the brain reduces pain. Decreased pain appears to be associated with a local increase in certain neurotransmitters within the nervous system, and the enkephalins in particular probably act as neurotransmitters activating serotonergic neurons, principally in the brain stem and medulla which, in their turn, play an important part in pain modulation at a spinal level. It will be clear to the reader that modulation of pain is not localised to one site in the nervous system and that interactions take place at several levels extending from the dorsal horns of the spinal cord through the thalamus to the limbic system and, perhaps, even to the cortex. These observations undoubtedly provide part of the explanation of why we are unable to control pain completely, why chronic pain is particularly difficult to suppress by pharmacological surgical or psychological means and why we often resort to a combination of two or more of these methods in an attempt to achieve pain relief.

Table 1 Intrinsic pain producing factors and their cells of origin

PPF	Cells of origin
5-hydroxytryptamine (Serotonin)	
Adenosine triphosphate (ATP)	Platelets
Potassium	
Adenosine phosphates (ATP, ADP, AMP)	Erythrocytes
Cationic protein in lysozymes	Leucocytes
Histamine	Mast cells
Hydrochloric acid	
Pepsin	Gastric cells
Kallikrein	
Trypsin	Pancreatic cells

CHEMICAL FACTORS WHICH PRODUCE PAIN

As long ago as 1914 von Frey concluded that nociceptor nerve endings are excited by physical stimuli only by the release of 'a chemical substance'. Sir Thomas Lewis in his classical work 'Pain' published in 1942 commented that: 'there is in normal skin a substance that is capable of giving rise to pain'. He also believed that the substance was not protein, potassium, histamine or acetylcholine although he knew all will cause pain if applied to subdermal tissues exposed by deroofing a blister. Later, as a result of experiments with artificially produced blister-base preparations, Professor Cyril Keele and his group suggested in 1950 that both bradykinin and serotonin (5-hydroxytryptamine) are in some way involved in pain generation. Both substances reduce the local threshold of pain sensitivity and cause local vasodilatation. In other words, they are vaso-neuroactive substances. Therefore, although there has been no difficulty in finding substances that will give rise to pain, there is uncertainty about which of them are actually released when tissue injury occurs and concerning the way in which they excite neuronal activity. It has become clear that pain receptors are chemoceptive. They may be stimulated by a variety of algesic agents, including hydrogen and potassium ions, some amines and peptides. Thus a specific chemical structure does not seem to be required for pain generation.

To summarise this complex and developing area, it appears that noxious stimuli give rise to pain as a result of the production or

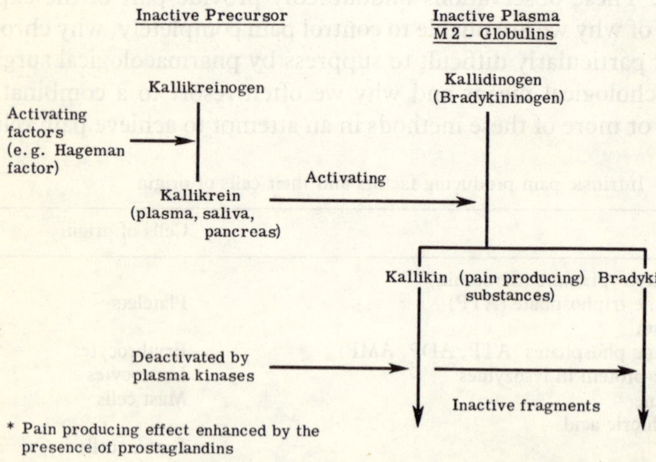

Fig 15. The activation of extrinsic plasma pain-producing substances

liberation of intrinsic chemical substances released by damaged cells (Table 1). These are algogenic, in other words they generate electrical activity in small diameter or C neurons directly, or activate other compounds to do so. Thus injury to tissues causes inflammation, oedema and pain because the intrinsic substances liberated from damaged cells in the area have a local effect causing vasodilatation, increased vascular permeability and pain. In addition, extrinsic factors, namely polypeptides known as kinins (kallidinogen and bradykinin) are formed in the plasma and a simplified diagram shows how they are activated (Fig. 15). These vaso-neuroactive substances may produce pain directly and certainly they increase sensitivity to noxious stimuli, for example by mechanical deformation. The effects are intensified by prostaglandins which are, themselves, generated by tissue damage.

Prostaglandins

Prostaglandins are long-chain fatty acids first discovered by the Swedish physiologist, von Euler, in 1934. He observed that extracts of seminal fluid cause vasodilatation and contraction in isolated intestine and the uterus. Von Euler believed that one substance produced by the prostate gland was responsible, (in fact it came from the seminal vesicles), and give it the name of prostaglandin. Almost 30 years later the chemical nature of prostaglandin was established and four related compounds were extracted from seminal fluid. They were labelled E_1, E_2, F_1 and F_2. Prostaglandins are derived from the essential fatty acid arachidonic acid which can be generated by all tissues so far investigated. More prostaglandins have been isolated in recent years and only certain ones appear to be involved in pain generation; they are PGE_2, $PGF_2\alpha$ and perhaps prostacyclin (Fig. 16). Their structure has been known for some time and the way in which they are derived from cell phospholipids via the arachidonic acid cascade is shown in Fig. 16. In 1971, a further significant event occurred when Dr John Vane, then of the Royal College of Surgeons of England and Nobel Prize winner in 1982 for his work on prostaglandins, demonstrated that aspirin and other non-corticosteroidal anti-inflammatory agents (NSAIAs) for example, indomethacin, mefenemates, phenylbutazone, etc. inhibited cyclo-oxygenase, which transforms arachidonate to various prostaglandins. It is also known that steroidal anti-inflammatory compounds (glucocorticoids) interfere with the production of prostaglandins by inhibiting the formation of accessible phospholipids—the step preceding the formation of arachidonic acid. It is not the purpose of

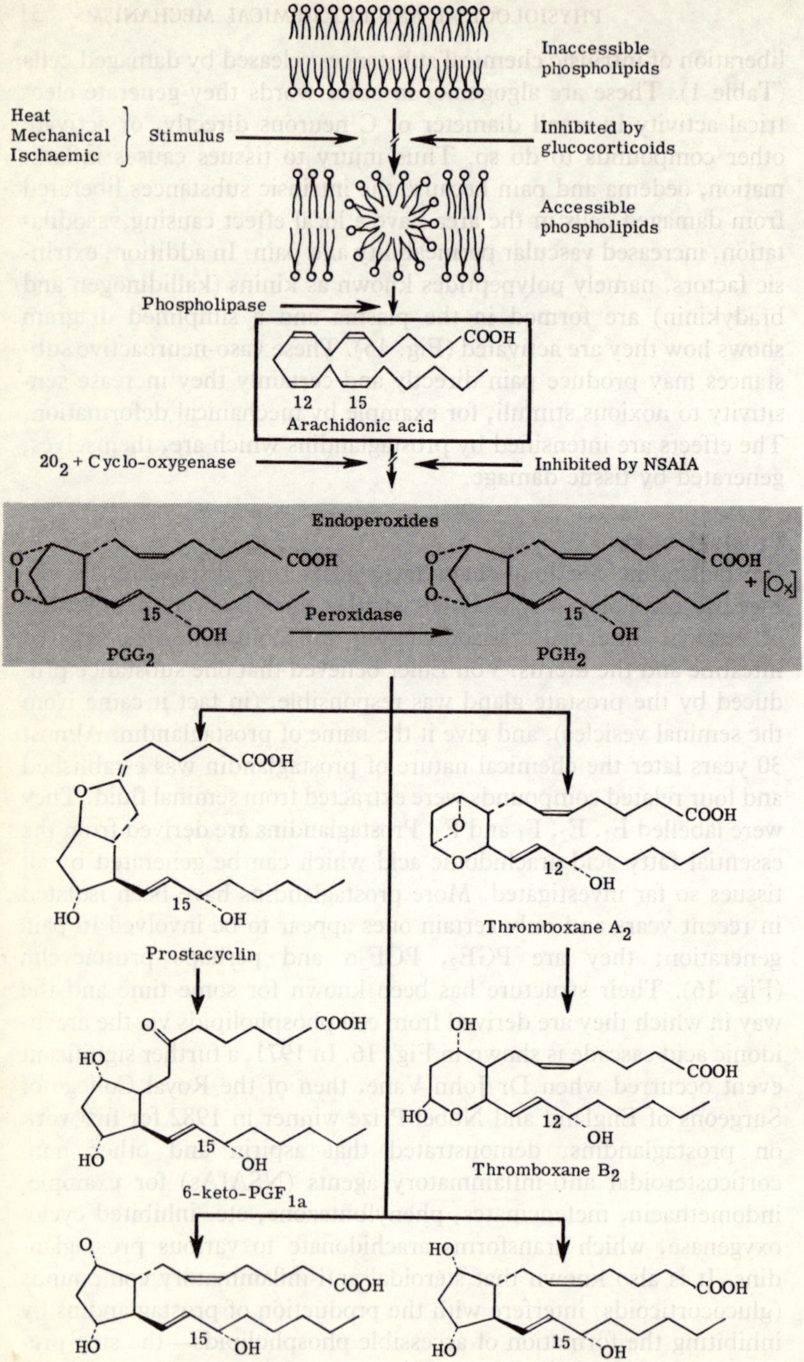

Fig 16. The prostaglandin cascade

Table 2 Possible role of the products of the arachidonic cascade in the production of pain and inflammation

Pain:	(Dolor)	Most products produce hyperalgesia. Pain is due to synergy with the kinins and histamine.
Heat: (Fever)	(Calor)	Caused by unknown arachidonic acid metabolites. NSAIAs and Aspirin are antipyretic.
Redness:	(Rubor)	Some products are potent vasodilators.
Swelling:	(Tumor)	Most products augment oedema induced by other agents — may simply reflect vasodilation.
Loss of function:	(Functiolaesa)	Products of the cascade have a potent effect on the movement and action of circulating inflammatory cells (platelets, PMNs, macrophages and lymphocytes).

Inflammation was defined as 'Rubor et tumor cum calore et dolore', by Cornelius Celsus (1st Cent), and 'et functiolaesa', was added by Rudolph Virchow (1882).

this book to deal with the nature of the entire range of actions of the prostaglandins but what is known of their role in the generation of inflammation, pain and fever, is summarised in Table 2.

3

The measurement of pain

'I often say that when you can measure what you are speaking about, and express it in numbers, you know something about it, but when you cannot measure it, when you cannot express it in numbers, your knowledge is of a meagre and unsatisfactory kind; it may be the beginning of knowledge, but you have scarcely, in your thoughts, advanced to the stage of science whatever the matter may be' (Lord Kelvin).

The fact that pain is a subjective phenomenon, and private to each of us, presents difficulties for those wishing to measure it, for how is it possible to estimate the extent of another's mental experiences? There are methods which, though they cannot tell us what is experienced when pain is felt, do give us information representing the subject's interpretation of the experience modified by what he or she wishes us to know about it. Alternatively we may evaluate a patient's pain in the light of our own experience or on the basis of observations we have made upon others in similar situations. When assessing pain we may, depending on our needs, measure sensitivity to induced pain in the laboratory or clinic or, on the other hand, measure the level of spontaneous pain caused by injury or disease.

The following aspects of pain measurement are described:

1. Pain thresholds.
2. Objective measurement of pain.
3. Subjective measurement of pain.
4. Indirect measurement of pain.

PAIN THRESHOLDS

Measurement of sensitivity to a noxious stimulus reveals the presence of two levels of response in all human beings. The first, known as the pain perception threshold, is reached when the quality of the experience produced by applying stimuli such as heat or pressure changes and pain is felt for the first time. The second, known as the severe pain threshold, is reached when the pain becomes unbearable on increasing the strength of the stimulus. Various stimuli have been used for this purpose, the chief ones being mechanical, electrical or thermal, and certain requirements must be met if the thresholds obtained are to be sufficiently reliable to enable us to relate them to other factors such as the effects of the environment, personality and ethnic background.

The characteristics of an ideal stimulus are as follows:

1. A range of power sufficient to reveal the thresholds described.
2. Accurate reproducibility.
3. Ease of control and safety in use. It should not cause excessive tissue damage.
4. A clearly defined quality which enables the subject to make an accurate assessment of threshold levels.

The two thresholds described are determined by physiological factors, but whereas there is relatively little difference between the values obtained for people of different social and ethnic groups for the lower one, values for the upper one vary widely and this seems to be due to combination of the effects of cultural and psychological factors. The interval between the thresholds is a measure of the degree of an individual's tolerance for pain. This varies widely, the variations being linked to personal and social factors. In general, both thresholds and tolerance are lower in women than in men and in more emotional people of either sex. They are also lower in those with emotional disorders characterised by anxiety, over-concern about health matters, or depression. Thresholds seem to be lower amongst clerical workers when compared with those who are in heavy manual work. In physical disease thresholds and levels of tolerance rise in some people but fall in others, the latter being characterised by a greater level of emotional disturbance. Thresholds are increased by analgesic drugs and by tranquillisers if anxiety is a marked feature of the condition. Interestingly, although pain thresholds are not increased in all but a few individuals by pharmacologically inert substances (placebos), such preparations relieve pain in about a third of those given them.

CLINICAL MEASUREMENT OF PAIN

Clinical assessment of pain usually involves an objective measurement by a doctor or nurse based upon the patient's comments, appearance and, significantly, upon the observer's own experience of pain and traditional cultural beliefs about the level of pain to be expected in any given illness. It involves the use of a 'word scale' and is open to a considerable degree of 'observer bias'. Therefore, increasing attention is now being paid to the use of subjective meas-

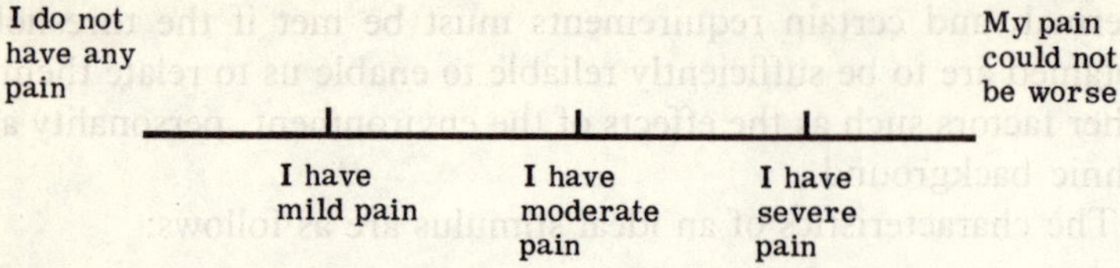

Fig 17. A simple verbal rating scale for pain measurement

ures of pain, which are preferred as they enable us to use the patient's own estimate of pain as a basis for treatment.

a. *The verbal rating scale*. Individuals are asked to rate their pain on a scale similar to one of those illustrated in Figure 17. The chief objection to these scales is that they provide only a coarse grading for pain. In addition the limitations of our language mean that the adjectives chosen give only a rough approximation of the experience. This difficulty was highlighted by the philosopher, Ludwig Wittgenstein, who wrote, 'For how can I go so far as to try to use language to get between pain and its expression'. As in all measures verbal scales are subject to the effects of personality and factors in the immediate environment. In order to reduce some of these objections other scales have been developed.

b. *The analogue scale*. As we are concerned with a subjective experience it seems more appropriate to provide the individual with a scale on which only the extremes of that experience appear allowing him or her to be freer in expressing pain by avoiding the use of other words. For this purpose an analogue scale is used as shown in Figure 18.

The analogue scale consists of a line 100 mm in length at the left hand end of which is printed, 'I do not have any pain', and at the right hand end, 'My pain could not be worse'. The patient is given the scale and asked to make a mark on the line at right angles to it at a point which represents the level of pain at the moment in question. The distance of the mark from the left end of the line is measured in millimetres and called a pain score. This is a measurement of pain intensity and in reality indicates what a patient wishes a doctor to know about the severity of his or her pain.

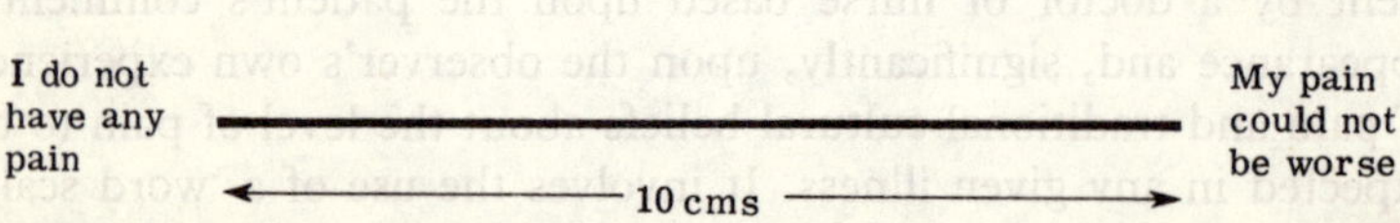

Fig 18. An analogue scale for pain measurement

If this process is repeated several times each day, or during a period of treatment of pain, the scores can be used to construct pain profiles from which the effectiveness of a treatment upon pain may be judged and an example of a pain profile is shown in Figure 19. This method, though simple, is not without difficulties, for example it cannot be used if the patient is confused and some elderly patients, and those of low intelligence, may not be able to master the technique. As with the verbal scales it is also open to the influences of personality, the effects of expectation by the doctor upon the patient's performance and various other factors in the immediate surroundings.

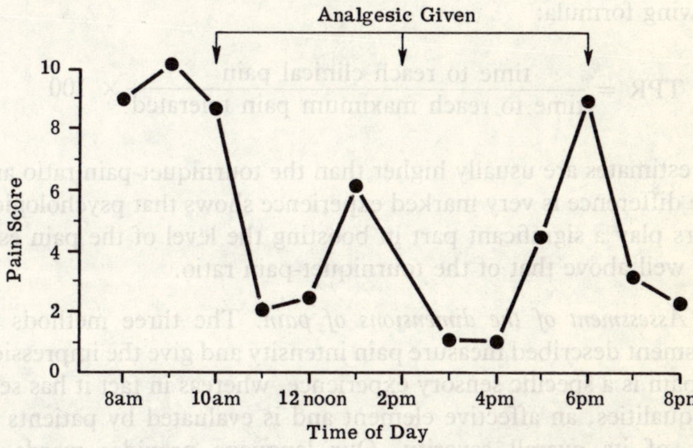

Fig 19. A pain profile showing responses to analgesic administration

c. *The pain estimate and tourniquet pain ratio.* Dr Richard Sternbach, an American psychologist, has described two methods for the assessment of pain. First, a pain estimate obtained by asking the patient to rate pain on a 0 to 100 scale using the following form of words: 'We need to get a more accurate idea of how severe your pain is. On a scale of 0 to 100 in which 0 is no pain at all, and 100 is pain so severe you would commit suicide if you had to endure it for more than a minute or two, what number would you give your average pain? What is your average pain these days?' This measure is meant to cover a period of hours and, though a useful rough check, it gives a much less detailed view of the fluctuations of pain throughout the day than the analogue scale which can be used as often as hourly or two-hourly. As the pain estimate may also be distorted by psychological and other factors, a second technique has been devised for use with it by which patients can compare spontaneous pain with artificially induced pain because it is believed that the production and reporting of the latter may be less subject to outside influences than the pain of disease or injury. In this method blood is first drained from the arm using an Esmarch or rubber bandage after which the state of limb ischaemia is maintained by the use of a pressure cuff on the upper arm set well above systolic blood pressure. The patient then squeezes a hand exerciser 20 times following which a stop watch is started and two times are recorded. The first is when pain reaches a level in the forearm similar to that caused by the illness or injury, and the second, the time taken to reach the maximum pain bearable. The tourniquet-pain ratio is then calculated from the following formula:

$$\text{TPR} = \frac{\text{time to reach clinical pain}}{\text{time to reach maximum pain tolerated}} \times 100$$

Pain estimates are usually higher than the tourniquet-pain ratio and if the difference is very marked experience shows that psychological factors play a significant part in boosting the level of the pain estimate well above that of the tourniquet-pain ratio.

d. *Assessment of the dimensions of pain.* The three methods of assessment described measure pain intensity and give the impression that pain is a specific sensory experience, whereas in fact it has sensory qualities, an affective element and is evaluated by patients in terms of its overall severity. Our language provides words to describe these three elements and Professor Ronald Melzack and others in Montreal have devised a pain questionnaire known as the 'McGill Pain Questionnaire' on the basis of this knowledge. They found that the words used to describe chronic pain may be categorised into the three groups mentioned and within each group words used also imply a certain level of pain. Table 3 shows some examples of the scales of words used to describe the sensory, affective and evaluative dimensions of pain and indicates the relative intensity value of each on a 5 point scale. (For full details of the McGill Pain Questionnaire the reader should consult 'Pain', volume 1, pages 277–299, 1975). From the full lists of words in the questionnaire, patients select those which best describe their pain and from these, measurements are derived giving information about both the quality of pain and its intensity. The questionnaire has been used to define the pain in different diseases more clearly and is sensitive enough to be used to assess the effectiveness of treatments for pain. In this situation it has the advantage of giving information about the influence of drugs upon the different dimensions of the pain experienced.

Table 3 Scales of words used to describe sensory, affective and evaluative dimensions of pain. Relative intensity value of each is indicated on a five-point scale.

	Sensory		Affective		Evaluative	
	Temporal	*Punctate, pressure*	*Fear*	*Punishment*		
1						1
2	flickering	pricking			annoying	2
	quivering	boring				
	pulsing	drilling			troublesome	
	throbbing					
3	beating				miserable	3
	pounding	stabbing	fearful	punishing		
		lancinating	frightful	gruelling	intense	
4			terrifying	cruel		4
				vicious	unbearable	
				killing		
5						5

The questionnaire has been translated into several languages in each of which national differences in the use of words to describe pain are encompassed.

INDIRECT CLINICAL MEASURES OF PAIN

Attempts have been made to indicate levels of pain by means of more indirect measurements. These techniques either depend upon the effect of pain on body function, or upon the amount of analgesic drug required to bring pain relief, or to bring it to a certain level. In the case of the former, severity of pain is linked with its effect upon respiratory vital capacity. This measure has been used post-operatively to assess the effect of analgesic drugs, and results are expressed as the in terms of a percentage of the pre-operative values. It has been suggested that vital capacity measurements are particularly valuable when assessing pain produced by abdominal and chest wall movement following thoracic or abdominal surgery.

4

The influence of learning and the environment on pain

In everyday medical practice knowledge of ways of measuring pain within and between individuals increases our ability to understand pain problems. However, it should be remembered that the earlier comments made about pain thresholds are based on studies of groups of people and that they do not always apply to any given individual although he or she has characteristics in terms of age, sex, social class and type of illness, in common with others who do fit the general pattern. Again, although measurements of pain are helpful when following a patient's progress under treatment, or when assessing the need for it, unexpected variations occur frequently and, for this reason, the many factors which influence pain must be considered when evaluating such measurements. The chief factors to be considered are:

1. The role of learning upon pain behaviour.
2. The effect of environmental factors upon pain.
3. Personality.
4. The meaning of pain.

THE ROLE OF LEARNING UPON PAIN BEHAVIOUR

We are not entirely certain that ability to experience pain and react to it is an inbuilt characteristic of man and animals. However, we are aware that, with rare exceptions, infants and very young children respond by withdrawing from a noxious stimulus and, if it is sufficiently severe, they grimace, cry and become pale and irritable. It is also common knowledge that within the first year or two of life children learn to avoid situations leading to pain and later come to express the nature of their experience with increasing sophistication in words. As childhood progresses the patterns of behaviour of the child in pain increasingly reflect family and wider cultural influences. For example, complaints of pain seem to be more frequent amongst the younger members of large families, amongst those from homes troubled by domestic strife where parents have quarrels and resort frequently to physical punishment of the child, and from homes where there is someone in the house who always has pain with associated emotional problems regarded by others as of 'a nervous kind'—in other words, in households where pain is part of someone's neurotic behaviour. Thus we believe that the withdrawal response to a noxious stimulus is innate and one upon which, through our own experience and observations of others in pain, we gradually build our repertoire of 'pain behaviour'. As will become evident later this is modified and moulded in its turn by more general factors in the environment and by our own emotional characteristics.

How do children view their pain? Such information is obviously important to those dealing with the ill child. One point is clear, a differentation in behaviour between boys and girls emerges early in life as boys develop the attitude expected by our society of males that they should be brave, although perhaps nervous or even afraid. By contrast girls are allowed to express their feelings more fully, although like boys they too grow to learn that to express emotion freely is not always tolerated. Fear of physical harm in certain circumstances is an obvious feature of childhood, especially amongst younger children and its presence seems to be important in determining the degree to which the child complains about pain. For example, a minor surgical procedure, such as an injection, may produce the most violent emotional upheaval if fear is prominent. This is in keeping with the fact that young children are upset by visible aspects of disease but unconcerned about lesions they cannot see. The consequences of illness do not seem to worry younger children; those less than eight or nine years of age are primarily concerned about being deprived of their play and when their pain disappears they seem to forget about it. Children of 10 years or more develop anxieties about the meaning of pain, the way in which their illness might cause loss of physical attractiveness, reduce their social activities or, if they are old enough, their career prospects. The angry feeling of 'Why should it be me?' is common amongst them and, in fact, the children of this age are beginning to show the emotional responses of adults to pain and illness. As childhood progresses control over emotion increases, but the effect of having experienced fear and controlled it shows in the pride with which children exhibit their scars and bruises to their peers and elders. Also, the child learns to recognise and complain about any disturbance of body function. It is during childhood too that the various meanings of pain are learned. The most obvious is the relation between pain and injury or disease, with the child also learning that pain may bring affection or be used to manipulate others; the need for the first and the use of the second are normal parts of our behaviour, but if incorporated in a major way in the development of relationships with others this may well lead to serious psychological difficulties in adolescence and adult life.

ETHNIC AND SOCIAL INFLUENCES UPON PAIN

Racial background has a powerful influence upon pain behaviour, although the ability to experience pain in response to noxious stimuli differs little between races. The differences show most obviously where tolerance of pain is concerned. For example, Northern and Western European races exhibit less emotion and complain less when in pain than Southern European or Latin races. In a study of pain amongst three racial groups in the United States individuals of old American stock, who are closest in their origins and general attitudes to native born British people, were noted to be phlegmatic and matter of fact about pain, whereas those of Italian origin complained more freely and emotionally about it, seeking treatment much sooner. Jewish people were found to behave in a similar manner openly seeking sympathy and support from relatives and friends which was readily given, and in fact there is reason to believe that this way of behaving does indeed help to relieve pain by reducing emotional tension. The factor governing behaviour for all groups seems to be the level of approval given for the public expression of pain and emotion. Unfortunately for those coming into a British society from a background where high levels of complaint are tolerated and, indeed, even expected, difficulties in gaining sympathy and treatment may be experienced and this should be remembered as the racial and cultural structure of the British Isles changes.

ENVIRONMENT AND ITS EFFECT UPON PAIN

External events around us affect both the severity of pain and behaviour associated with it. Intense and prolonged focussing of attention on activities associated with a high level of physical and emotional involvement may prevent the appearance of pain, as for example in a football match where a kick or blow passes unnoticed until the heat of the moment is passed. In wartime, soldiers, though seriously wounded, may not feel pain at all and fight on until a lull in the battle occurs. It is known that the need for powerful narcotic drugs amongst the seriously wounded is low or even non-existent in many instances, although demands for them are much higher amongst civilians with similar injuries. This is because the circumstances of the injury are important because, for soldiers wounding means withdrawal from battle and a reduced chance of sudden death making the wounds almost desirable, but in the case of civilians anxiety about the physical and social consequences of injury are considerable as they may present a threat to an individual's whole way of life. The injury to them may be a catastrophe. Doctors encounter these patterns of behaviour amongst their patients quite frequently. Thus, injury or disease with long-term consequences, including loss of physical wellbeing and strength, loss of earning power, and loss of family and social status, is associated with anxiety at first, often anger and resentment too, and then depression and reduced ability to tolerate pain. If physical incapacity is short-lived and known to be remediable, however unpleasant, it produces a different response. There is still initial anxiety and heightened preoccupation with the body, but ability to bear pain is greater and depression does not occur so often.

It is not only the significance of illness or injury that produces emotional changes. The attitudes of others, especially doctors and nurses, have a very powerful effect upon the sufferer and, although generally these effects are beneficial, sometimes they provoke anxiety, fear and uncertainty, and occasionally frank resentment or hostility. Emotional tensions of this kind are usually aroused when patients feel that their problems are not being taken seriously enough, where doctors seem to be in doubt about diagnosis or treatment and where they feel, rightly or wrongly, that medical or nursing staff are antagonistic towards them. The latter situation may arise because of traditional views about pain, mentioned earlier, and the medical staff's view of how patients 'should behave' when in pain. Unfortunately men appear to suffer most, for it is believed,

Table 4 The pattern of administration of analgesic drugs to men and women in Radiotherapy wards*

	Men	Women
Number of patients	15	12
Number of occasions drugs given at patient's request	23	28
Number of occasions drugs given on initiative of nurses	1	22
Number of occasions on which nurses refused patient's request for drugs	18	0

* Drugs requested and given during one week.

in Britain at least, that they should bear pain with little complaint as illustrated by the figures in Table 4. If they do not do so they may find that drugs are not easily obtained and, when given, are relatively ineffective; signs that doctors and nurses are punishing patients, unconsciously or otherwise, for their 'bad behaviour'. Where nurses have been taught to understand patients' pain and deal with it by physical and psychological means, patients express a much greater degree of satisfaction with their treatment than where the staff have not received any training of this kind. It is also worth noting that in hospital wards nursing sisters are the key figures in a patient's appeal for pain relief because their attitudes colour those of the rest of the nursing staff and therefore the atmosphere of the ward and the patients' emotional wellbeing. By contrast doctors, especially more senior ones, are regarded as more remote and detached, though interested people.

5

Personality and pain

Personality is that blend of intellectual and emotional qualities reflected in our behaviour and unique to each individual, yet possessing a basic structure the essential elements of which may be measured. In people of normal intelligence intellect plays a far less important role in the experience of pain than emotion, which consequently forms the centre of interest for those studying psychological aspects of pain. The value of a knowledge of a patient's personality prior to his or her developing a painful illness, or pain without evidence of organic disease, must be emphasised both for its use as a baseline from which to estimate the degree of change that occurs in the individual as a result of pain, and to enable one to predict how he or she will behave when in pain and respond to treatment, whether physical, psychological, or some combination of both. A knowledge of a patient's personality also tells us something of their ways of coping with stresses and strains in life, their liability to emotional breakdown and, therefore, the likelihood of their dealing effectively with a chronically painful disorder, the prospect of mutilation by surgery, or even of death in a terminal illness. Personality may be examined from the clinical standpoint by dividing individuals into groups which demonstrate common characteristics of emotion known as 'personality traits'. Those which are important in the understanding of pain are:

1. Proneness to anxiety.
2. Proneness to depression.
3. Hysterical traits.
4. Hypochondriacal traits.
5. Obsessional traits.

A number of the traits listed (1–4) merge into emotional disorders which are often associated with complaints of pain (see page 134). An alternative way of looking at personality and pain is to relate them through the measurement of each factor. After the characteristics of the various emotional traits mentioned and their influence upon pain have been described, two methods of measuring personality will be discussed.

PERSONALITY TRAITS

Anxiousness

The anxious person is one who responds to everyday and unavoidable stresses of life by worrying about them, though more stable individuals would remain unperturbed in similar circumstances. This tendency is linked with uncertainty and apprehension in new situations which may well be avoided if tension becomes too great. Illness, especially if severe, chronic, or uncertain in its outcome, will inevitably raise levels of anxiety in most people, but to the anxiety prone person it may become a considerable burden and evoke levels of emotion requiring professional medical treatment. Whether this state is reached or not pain will be greater for patients who have a tendency to become anxious because pain causes anxiety and, in its turn, anxiety heightens pain.

Depressiveness and the cyclothymic personality

Feelings of low spiritedness are familiar to almost everyone and occur from time to time as a normal feature of our responses to certain kinds of stress, especially disappointments, failures and losses of various kinds. Some are able to bear their troubles with considerable fortitude, but others feel despair quickly and respond in this way to what might seem a quite trivial matter to the emotionally more equable person. It may be that the individual who is prone to become depressed is at other times happy-go-lucky, carefree and high spirited, or even elated, in which case they are regarded as having a 'cyclothymic' personality, being a person of changing moods. Fortunately in most cyclothymic people the optimistic cheerful element of the personality predominates. Pain, especially if chronic, brings feelings of depression and those who become depressed easily may not only sink emotionally, but simultaneously experience more pain if it happens to be present for any reason. At the same time they show reduced ability to cope with it.

Hysterical traits

It is said that hysterical traits are most often found amongst members of the theatrical profession, and others who seek and enjoy the limelight in the everyday world. Individuals with an hysterical personality show immaturity in their emotions and behaviour. They are dramatic, extraverted, and shallow in their affections, transferring them freely from one person to another. They seek excitement, dress for effect, and enjoy emotional scenes in which they express themselves freely and from which they may emerge with a sense of righteous indignation or no obvious discomfort, whereas the other person involved feels exhausted and drained of all emotion. These episodes may well arise from the hysteric's sensitivity to the remarks of others, perhaps unintentionally made, and their quickness to take offence. When in pain the individual with this trait, usually a woman, exaggerates symptoms, becoming evermore demanding and manipulative, and tolerating pain poorly. This often brings them into conflict with a doctor or nurse whose expectations of how patients 'should' behave results in tensions that heighten quickly, sometimes leading to a breaking of the patient's relationship with the medical staff. On the other hand, the patient's tensions and apparent affections for the doctor, also freely shown, may cause him to feel considerable embarrassment.

'Hysterics', which are sudden, massive, and uncontrolled eruptions of emotion, are not necessarily shown by people with hysterical personalities and occur in response to some overwhelming stress, usually emotional and seldom physical in origin. Hysterical conversion symptoms are described on page 141.

Hypochondriacal traits

It is normal for most medical students to imagine at some stage of their career that they have the symptoms of an illness for which there is inadequate evidence. Most cope with such anxieties without visiting the local student Health Clinic, but a few do not and seek reassurance. A tendency to worry about health matters in this way from time to time is regarded as normal amongst medical students, but preoccupation with body functions expressed in terms of constant and excessive efforts to keep fit in a way that is out of keeping with one's age group, unremitting worries about some aspects of bodily function, and the frequent use of patent medicines or visits to the doctor's surgery with a series of trivial complaints, suggests the existence of hypochondriacal traits. Aches and pains are common among such folk who generally require little other than reassurance to remove their symptoms. Excessive numbers of clinical investigations and the prolonged use of medicines are counter-productive with them and powerful drugs of any kind should be avoided. As may be imagined, one of the problems faced by the doctor who has such a patient is determining whether or not the symptoms have an organic cause and need physical treatment; a situation in which knowledge of the patient's past medical and social history together with elicitation of a careful history of symptoms are mandatory if difficulties are to be avoided.

Obsessional traits

Punctuality, reliability, a high moral tone, opposition to change, the need for routine, and a tendency to meticulousness, are characteristic of the person with an obsessional personality type. The need for orderliness, abhorrence of uncertainty and seeing the world as only black or white without shades of grey can make treatment of any physical illness, especially one which is painful, an ordeal for the doctor who is constantly asked for more information than he can give about causes, about treatments that produce symptom relief without side effects, and about precise details of the future which he cannot give, especially in a chronic illness. He is most likely to succeed in coping with such a patient if he is truthful and as concise in his opinion as possible, giving good reasons for his inability to answer questions completely. Evasiveness will not be tolerated and neither will any evidence that the doctor has not carefully checked all aspects of diagnosis and treatment at each stage. Needless to say such conditions are not easy to keep and tensions or hostility may arise in the patient, the doctor, or both as a result!

MEASUREMENT OF PERSONALITY

Basic personality attributes may be measured in several ways and two of these have been chosen to illustrate the value of formal personality assessment. They are:

1. The Eysenck personality inventory (EPI).
2. The Minnesota multiphasic personality inventory (MMPI),

The Eysenck personality inventory

The Eysenck Personality Inventory, developed by Professor Hans Eysneck and Dr S. G. Eysenck, measures two dimensions of personality regarded as fundamental because they are related directly to physiological activity of the central nervous system. The dimensions are stability/neuroticism (N) and introversion/extraversion (E). Measurement of the former gives an estimate of an individual's degree of emotionality and, in particular, liability to breakdown in a neurotic manner when under stress. The higher a person's N score the greater the emotional vulnerability shown. A higher score does not necessarily mean that the individual is neurotic or suffering from a disorder of emotional life, it merely denotes a level of susceptibility to breakdown greater than that of those who make lower scores. An extravert is a person with an outgoing personality and the greater the score on the E scale the more an individual will be found to be gregarious and cheerful with high levels of energy and a constant need for stimulation. The introvert by contrast tends to be solitary, relatively uncommunicative, serious minded, and uncomfortable in large gatherings. Both personality dimensions have a significant relation to pain threshold measurements. In general terms thresholds for pain, especially the upper or severe pain threshold, are lower for introverts than for extraverts. However, clinical observations show that extraverts complain much more freely than introverts, although they have higher pain thresholds. With regard to measures of neuroticism, those who make high scores have most pain. Therefore, as experience of pain is greatest in the introverts with high neuroticism scores and lowest in stable extraverts, why should clinical experience be at variance with laboratory findings with regard to pain thresholds? One explanation for the discrepancy was revealed in a study of the relation between pain and complaint behaviour and personality amongst women in childbirth. It was found that the more extraverted women reported their labour pains as greater than the introverts, a fact that was confirmed by nurses' observations. Therefore, it was concluded that extraverts have a greater tendency to exaggerate their feelings and that this dominates the clinical situation.

The Minnesota personality inventory

The MMPI is more popular in the United States than in Britain. It is a lengthy questionnaire which has 14 scales of measurement providing a wide profile of personality attributes. For this reason it has considerable appeal but, as administration may take up to two hours, it is less attractive for use in the seriously ill than EPI, which can be completed in 10 to 15 minutes. As in the case of the EPI the MMPI is a checklist of physical and emotional symptoms, including both those from the past and those present at the time of examination. High scores on the various items indicate the presence of an emotional disturbance and patterns of scores typical for acute and chronic painful illnesses have been identified. These are known as 'profiles of personality'. Thus for patients with chronic pain significantly higher scores are found on those items measuring hypochondriasis (Hs), depression (D) and hysteria (Hy). This is shown in Figure 20. By contrast, patients with acute pain show high scores for hypochondriasis (Hs) and hysteria (Hy), but not for depression (D). These differences indicate that acute and chronic pain bring

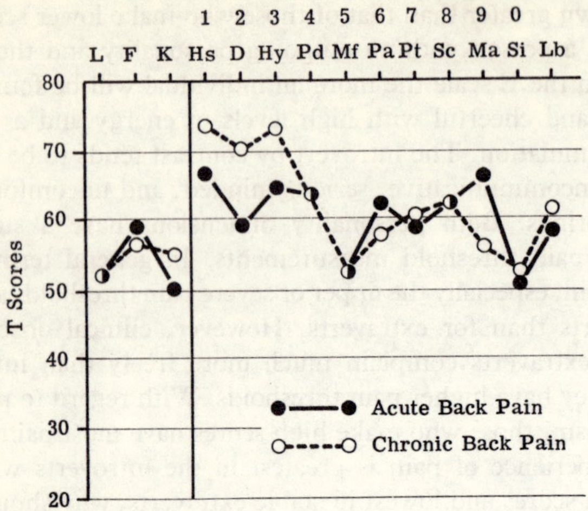

Fig 20. Personality profiles obtained using the Minnesota Multiphasic Personality Inventory (MMPI) (from Sternbach, R.A. 1973)

preoccupation with bodily function, but perhaps because of the level of this preoccupation and tendency of people with an acute illness to express agitation, reflected in the mania scale (Ma), depressive feelings are less apparent amongst them. In a chronic painful illness the amount of concern about the body increases (Hs and Hy), depression becomes more obvious (D) and the level of agitation falls (Ma).

One of the main attractions of the MMPI is that personality profiles permit the identification of certain groups of characteristics on the basis of which the patients with pain problems may be 'typed'. For example, they may be found to belong to the depressive, hypochondriacal or hysterical group, the general characteristics of which in each case are in keeping with the personality traits described earlier.

6

The meaning of pain

We accept that pain indicates damage to some part of our body, and that the complaints of others in pain indicate their level of suffering. Some are aware from their own experiences that a pain may be used to attract more attention, love or affection, than can be justified by its true intensity and, furthermore, that at times pain is used as a means of manipulating others or gaining control over them. It is seldom appreciated, however, that pain may develop as a means of causing the person concerned to suffer, not because physical damage is present, but because the suffering seems necessary to relieve guilt about some earlier event in life, or even about thoughts which have raised guilty feelings. At times pain also serves to reduce intense feelings of loss, for example, it may be the substitute for such feelings in mourning, or for loss of part of the body, as after amputation of a limb. Therefore the significance of pain varies, that is, it may be symbolic of problems of both a physical and emotional kind. Three types of symbolisation have been identified and they are as follows:

1. Pain as evidence of physical damage.
2. Pain as a means of communication.
3. Pain as a means of manipulating others, expressing hostility, or relieving guilt.

It has been suggested by Professor George Engel, an American psychiatrist, that there are certain individuals for whom the presence of pain is essential for the prevention or relief of emotional turmoil. They are called 'pain-prone people'. The pain of which they complain is usually without an obvious organic cause and is therefore known as 'psychogenic pain'. A pain-prone person is characterised by a pessimistic, gloomy and depressive personality. Somehow they always seem to be unsucessful or unlucky in the lottery of life, but on closer examination of the causes of their misfortunes it appears that they are usually instrumental themselves in bringing them about. They are at their best emotionally when behaving stoically in the face of genuine physical illness and yet paradoxically seem to develop pain just when success appears to be within their grasp. Such individuals could be regarded as masochistic because their behaviour is self-punitive and it should be remembered that the relationship between pain and punishment has been established for a long time, as indicated by its roots in Latin (*poena*) and Greek (*poine*), each meaning penalty or punishment. Looking back over the lives of pain-prone people, feelings of aggression and suffering are prominent amongst them, and resentment against doctors is a marked feature of their contact with the medical profession.

Dr Thomas Szasz has also drawn attention to a pain-prone type of individual who he called 'homo dolorosus', and to whom he attributed the following characteristics:

1. Chronic, intractable or unbearable pain, which is a sign that the sufferer wishes to occupy the sick role. In the absence of an organic cause this is the hallmark of 'homo dolorosus'.
2. The patient's identity and social role are verified by pain and suffering in the same way that a doctor's identity and social role are verified by his medical qualifications.
3. 'Homo dolorosus', having established a role as a 'professional in pain', engages in 'painmanship', a way of feeling and behaving which is characterised by the presence of undiagnosable pain and unrelievable suffering, yet creating meaning for life and power to control the environment. Naturally this poses a great challenge to the doctor's professional skills and identity which rests primarily on his ability to diagnose illness and relieve pain and suffering. If he is defeated by the patient's symptoms on several occasions he begins to formulate more and more obscure diagnoses and performs unnecessary surgical or other investigatory and therapeutic activities which may well be to the patient's physical disadvantage, although supporting him in his unconsciously chosen role. On the other hand the doctor may reject the patient and discharge him from further care.
4. Having established an abnormal way of life, 'homo dolorosus' seldom relinquishes the role and its gains, demanding frequent medical and surgical attention to maintain the status quo. It is, therefore, to be expected that such individuals reject offers of psychological investigation, usually by presenting fresh physical symptoms. It is not surprising that they arouse antagonistic and unsympathetic feelings in relatives and friends, and especially in doctors, and other medical professionals in contact with them.

Although the ideas about symbolism just described, and the use of pain to gain relief from emotional stresses, are questioned on the grounds that they are unproven scientifically, many clinicians feel from their personal experience that they are quite acceptable. However, the number of those who are pain-prone people, or who qualify for the title 'homo dolorosus' is very small when seen against the vast numbers of patients with pain problems. An account of their characteristics draws attention in a rather dramatic way to the necessity for doctors to be aware of their relationships with patients, especially if they have chronic pain, because this is when the meaning of the symptoms may differ for each. Normally the ill person takes up what is called the 'sickness role'. This is a state granted to the individual by society which expects him or her to report illness as unacceptable and expects that every effort should be made to collaborate with doctors and other medical personnel. In addition, the sick are expected to use all the resources made available to them by society in order to get well as quickly as possible. Whilst occupying the sick role the ill person is freed from the usual responsibilities of life at home and at work and as long as there seems to be a genuine physical basis for illness society accepts occupancy of the role. However, there are occasions on which it rejects the latter and then patients are said to be exhibiting 'abnormal illness behaviour'.

As indicated earlier illness is not always unwelcome because some people find the protection it gives them against the stresses produced by the responsibilities of everyday life rewarding. At the same time the doctor, family or friends, may begin to feel that the ill person is prolonging his or her illness unreasonably and having broken the rules of society they are regarded as behaving abnormally. Some develop this style of behaviour when a child as a consequence of pain experienced at that time, but others do not do so until the appearance of a painful illness or injury in adult life when they learn that unmet emotional needs, such as the need for affection, can be fulfilled by the maintenance of the sickness role, or where abnormal behaviour is reinforced by full or partial satisfaction of such needs. However, it should be remembered that those from lower social economic groups, especially if they have had a poor education, tend to present emotional difficulties in the form of somatic symptoms. Readjustment of a person's view of the relation between emotional events and complaints of physical distress, especially pain should, in the light of this comment, reduce the chances of an incorrect diagnosis. The results of failure to recognise this association lead to difficulty because when abnormal illness behaviour develops the relationship between the doctor and the patient often changes and if the latter does not have insight into the patient's difficulties, or if he or she does not have the skills or inclination to deal with them a complete breakdown in communication between the two may occur. The doctor may then label the patient 'neurotic' or 'hysterical' whilst the patient regards the doctor as a failure.

The following examples illustrate two common situations in which the abnormal sickness role was employed for gain, which in the first case was monetary gain and, in the second, a ready supply of powerful analgesic drugs.

Case 1. The first patient was a middle-aged married man who had a simple manual job. He suffered a trivial injury to his head during the course of his work and within days developed headaches, visual disturbances and generalised weakness. His family doctor suggested a spell away from work, but to his dismay found that the man's symptoms, and in particular his headaches, persisted for weeks and months. Compensation was sought at an early stage, but throughout his time away from work the patient gave the impression to all who examined him medically that he was very anxious to resume his job. His family accepted him as a sick person and fostered this role, as did the doctors who saw him initially reinforcing the situation with unnecessary investigations and indecision about the true nature of his problems. Eventually a psychiatric examination was carried out and the patient was told that he did not have a serious physical disorder and was advised to return to work which, after some time, he did. The investigation of his past revealed similar episodes and on each occasion the abnormal sickness role was maintained for monetary gain.

Case 2. The second patient was a man who had a history of chronic peptic ulcer symptoms for which he underwent surgical treatment. Within a short time he began to experience recurrent bouts of severe abdominal pain for which he was given powerful analgesics. On several occasions the pain was sufficiently severe to merit further abdominal explorations. No satisfactory organic basis was found for the pain and only after several years of investigations involving frequent differences of opinion with the surgeons involved, was it realised that the man was addicted to his analgesic drugs, the power of which had increased as time passed. Ultimately, the situation was exposed and treatment for addiction was carried out. In this case prolongation of the sickness role enabled the patient to continue taking powerful analgesics 'legitimately'. He evaded the issue of addiction for several years by firmly maintaining his role as a surgical patient with a chronic pain problem. He was so successful that surgeons continued to accept his challenge to them to find a source for the pain which they sought to do only on the basis that it must be organic, which was precisely what the patient wished.

MASOCHISM AND SADISM

Masochism and sadism refer to forms of perverted behaviour, especially sexual behaviour. In the case of the former the sufferer, and in the latter the one who is inflicting the suffering, derive pleasure and sexual arousal from experiencing or giving pain or humiliation. The word masochism is derived from the name of Leopold Sacher-Masoch, a 19th century writer whose works describe this form of eroticism. Sadism is derived from the name of 18th century French writer, Marquis de Sade, who was at one time sentenced to death for his sexual cruelty. Having evaded death he escaped and later wrote romantic novels, but eventually became insane. Masochism and sadism are quite common in mild degrees and when present often occur together in the same individual to a variable extent.

PART TWO

Clinical analysis of pain

7

General characteristics of pain

At first sight consideration of how people describe pain may seem unimportant, but a moment's reflection reveals that accounts of pain tell us two things about it. First, the nature of pain due to a specific condition tends to be described similarly by different individuals, thus its qualities seem to be unique. Second, the vividness of the description given is related to a person's emotional constitution, his cultural and ethnic background, and the significance of the pain. In clinical practice great emphasis is placed in the location of pain and the qualities which enable the physician or surgeon to ascribe its origin to a particular organ or part of the body. For example, the pain of myocardial infarction is typically described as heavy or crushing and as a sensation which grips the chest as though in a vice. Sciatica, which is due to compression of lumbar or sacral nerve roots by a prolapsed intervertebral disc, is regarded as being like an electric shock, or a stab in the buttock, which radiates to the knee or foot. The words chosen give a good indication of the pain's severity and it has been shown that there is a range of adjectives upon which we draw when describing the various sensory and emotional qualities of pain, but it should be remembered that these differ from one part of the country to another.

Cutaneous pain

The skin has a wider variety of sensory nerves than any other organ of the body and therefore damage to it is located more accurately and described with greater precision than elsewhere. If the skin alone is involved the words cutting or burning are often used, but if blood vessels are contributing to the pain it becomes throbbing in nature. When damage to nerve fibre endings in the skin takes place this gives rise to itching, tingling, smarting or stinging pains, and with damage to larger fibres in mixed nerves the pain becomes sharper or brighter. If abnormalities develop during the process of repair in major nerves a very unpleasant burning pain may follow in its area of distribution and this is known as causalgia.

Deep somatic pain

Pain due to acute disorders of joints is well localised and usually described as sharp and burning, or throbbing. In more chronic conditions, though well localised, dull aching pains are experienced upon which movement superimposes stabbing or lancinating pain. Bone pain is not so well localised and arises from stimulation of nerve fibres in the periosteum. It is described as a deep soreness or aching and if inflammation is present it takes on a throbbing quality. Similarly muscle pain is poorly localised and is described as a dull ache or a cramp. Thus, the sensitivity of the structures described and others related to them varies; periosteum is the most sensitive tissue followed in order by ligaments, fibrous corpuscles, joints, tendons, and fasciae. The bodies of muscles are the least sensitive of all.

Visceral pain

The pleura, pericardium and peritoneum are in constant movement themselves and enclose organs which are mobile. All are supplied with small diameter nerve fibres and when stimulated, for example by the products of inflammation, are a source of severe pain which varies in intensity with movement, and is described as stabbing, lancinating, sharp or cutting, cramping or crushing. The gut is a source of either a gnawing or cramping pain, or the intermittent pain known as colic when irritated by chemical substances produced by inflammation following perforation or when distended. Other distensible structures within the abdomen, for example the gallbladder, common bile duct and ureters, also give rise to colic. In the case of the urinary bladder obstruction to outflow produces distension and a sensation of crushing or bursting pain which may become extreme and unbearable. Studies of the sensitivities of various viscera and allied tissues shows that parietal serous membranes are the most sensitive followed by the walls of hollow viscera and parenchymatous organs. It is important to remember that noxious stimulation of viscera for example, the ureter or renal pelvis leads to contraction of muscles of the abdominal wall supplied by the same spinal segments. This is known as a visceromotor reflex and it is responsible for the phenomenon of 'muscle guarding'—an important clinical sign of visceral inflammation. Similar reflex activity produces rigidity and tenderness in muscles around inflamed joints together with hyperalgesia of overlying skin.

Ischaemic pain

Pain arising from heart muscle as the result of ischaemia is described as a constricting sensation, or as a cramping or crushing and, in addition, because of the emotive nature of the situation, adjectives like terrifying or horrifying may be added.

Pain arising from the nervous system

Disorders of the brain and spinal cord give rise to pain by compressing peripheral or sensory nerves prior to their entry into the central nervous system, by stretching the dura mater as happens when there is an expanding intracranial mass, or its distension by dilatation of blood vessels within it. Pressure or traction upon the dura mater gives rise to an aching pain of a generalised nature which, if due to vascular dilatation, has a beating or throbbing quality.

Examination of patients with pain

The examiner must first take a careful history of a painful disorder, including a detailed account of its mode of onset, nature, distribution, and response to physical and emotional events. At this stage the description of pain and its development may make it possible to reach a diagnosis. However, further information should be gained to support this by appropriate examination of the part of the body affected. During the course of the examination other characteristics of pain behaviour become evident. Thus, pain changes behaviour and assessments of severity are dependent both on what is said about it and also upon non-verbal, facial and bodily indicators too. For example, at times of severe pain accompanying signs include sweating, increased respiratory rate, skin pallor, and even vomiting. Patients exhibit changes in emotion with apprehension, panic or even terror, they may become solitary and depressed or exhibit raised levels of emotional tension with accompanying outbursts of irritability and intolerance of others around them.

Until recently agreement upon the terms to be used to describe various aspects of pain had not been reached but in 1979 the International Association for the Study of Pain issued a list of pain terms which it is hoped will become accepted throughout the world. The glossary is meant to provide a *minimum standard vocabulary* for clinicians and as such represents a carefully selected battery of words from those available.

Pain terms	*Definition*
Pain:	An unpleasant sensory and emotional experience associated with actual or potential tissue damage, or described in terms of such damage
Allodynia:	This is a new term which should be given to pain arising as a result of *non-noxious* stimulations of *normal skin*. For example,

	non-noxious stimulation of skin may give rise to pain at the site of referred pains.
Analgesia:	Absence of pain to noxious stimulation.
Anaesthesia Dolorosa:	Pain in an area which is anaesthetic.
Causalgia:	A syndrome of sustained burning pain after a traumatic nerve lesion combined with vasomotor and sudomotor dysfunction and late trophic changes.
Central Pain:	Pain associated with a lesion of the central nervous system, e.g. infarctions of the thalamus, or in cases of multiple sclerosis.
Dysaesthesia:	An *unpleasant abnormal sensation* whether spontaneous or not. (See Parasthesia).
Hyperalgesia:	Increased sensitivity to *noxious* stimulation. This is the result of a lowered threshold to noxious stimulation.
Hyperaesthesia:	Increased sensitivity to stimulation, excluding special senses but including other modes of cutaneous sensitivity including touch and thermal sense without pain.
Hyperpathia:	A painful *syndrome*, characterised by delayed pain over-reaction and after-sensation to a stimulus, especially a repetitive stimulus. It may be associated with hypo- or hyperaesthesia, or dysaesthesia.
Hypoalgesia:	Diminished senstivity to *noxious* stimulation.
Hypoaesthesia:	Decreased sensitivity to stimulation, excluding special senses.
Neuralgia:	Pain in the distribution of a nerve or nerves. It is a term that should *not* be reserved only for paroxysmal pains.
Neuropathy:	A disturbance of function or pathological change in a nerve or in several nerves.
Neuritis:	A special form of neuropathy reserved for inflammatory processes affecting nerves.
Nociceptor:	A receptor preferentially sensitive to a noxious or potentially noxious stimulus.
Noxious:	A noxious stimulus is a tissue damaging stimulus.
Paraesthesia:	An *abnormal sensation* whether spontaneous or evoked (see Dysaesthesia).
Pain threshold:	The least stimulus intensity at which a subject perceives pain.

Pain tolerance level: The greatest stimulus intensity causing pains that a subject is prepared to tolerate.

This glossary is a slightly shortened form of the full version published in Pain, vol. 6, pp. 249–252 (1979).

A SIMPLE PAIN ANALYSIS QUESTIONNAIRE

In full analysis of pain problems the following series of questions should be asked about the pain:

Location

1. Where does it hurt?
2. Is the site of your pain constant or does it move and if so to where and under what circumstances?

Onset

3. When did your pain start? (Hours, days, weeks, months, years).
4. Did your pain begin suddenly, or gradually?
5. Can you remember the event, or events, which appeared to produce your pain when it began?

Course

6. Is your pain present
   a. throughout the day,
   b. part of every day (specify),
   c. part of every week (specify),
   d. occasionally, each month, or less often than that (specify),
   e. at night, and does it interrupt sleep?

Character

7. How would you describe your pain?
8. How strong is your pain? Please tell me which of the following words describes it most nearly—mild, discomforting, distressing, horrible, excruciating (this is only one of several verbal scales that might be used).
9. Does your pain worsen with
   a. movement or changes in posture, e.g. standing, sitting, lying, bending,
   b. coughing, sneezing or straining,
   c. eating or drinking?
10. Will any of the following relieve your pain—rest, sleep, changes in posture, e.g. standing, sitting, lying or bending?

Effects of pain

11. Does your pain interfere with
    a. normal activities in the home,
    b. normal activities at work,
    c. normal social activities in any way?

Effects of emotion

12. a. Does your pain lessen or increase when you are worried, tense or depressed?
    b. Does your pain lessen when you are enjoying yourself, or when you are busy?

Effects of specific treatment

What is the effect of any of the following forms of treatment you may have had upon your pain?

Drugs

1. Pain killers (analgesics).
2. Drugs for nervous tension (minor or major tranquillisers).
3. Drugs for sleep (hypnotics).
4. Drugs for depression (anti-depressants).
5. Other drugs, including preparations for specific conditions associated with pain, such as antacids and antispasmodics in stomach and bowel disorders, anti-inflammatory agents in disorders of joints, anti-migraine preparations and local applications of rubefacients, (counter-irritants).
6. Alcohol.

Physical and psychological treatments

1. Physiotherapy, i.e. exercises, local heat and massage.
2. Surgical treatments, including injections of local anaesthetics or steroid preparations, nerve section, cordotomy, and manipulation.
3. Acupuncture.
4. Hypnosis, or other psychological treatments.

REGIONAL PAIN

In Chapters 8, 9 and 10 clinical features of a number of common painful conditions are described together with a brief notes on treatment and comment upon their relation to emotion where appropriate.

8

Headache, facial, neck and eye pain

Headache is perhaps one of the commonest afflictions of everyday life and few people have not experienced it. The structures of the face and head are richly innervated by sensory, motor and autonomic nerves. The sensations of sight, hearing, taste and smell are received here, and the face and voice being vehicles of emotion and communication are very significant to us. Thus, this part of the body, where much of our contact with the outside world takes place, is a likely area for both organic and psychologically induced pain and, in fact the latter occurs in and around the head and neck more often than in any other area.

MUSCLE TENSION HEADACHE

The development of a headache is a common response to stressful events and the pain, usually described as being 'like a band around the head' or, 'pressure on top of the head', or, tightness in the region of the temples or back of the head, is due to increased muscle tension most probably stimulating nerve endings in the muscular aponeuroses. Pain in the temporal region is due to temporalis muscle spasm and arises in individuals who, under stress, clench their jaws tightly for long periods, an action which also gives rise to facial pain as the same movements involve increasing tension in the masseter and pterygoid muscles. Headache arising as a result of muscle tension varies in duration from a matter of minutes to weeks. Often the scalp is tender on palpation and there are complaints of neck stiffness. Acute pain may be elicited on palpation of small areas or 'trigger spots' in one or more of the following muscles—trapezius, sternomastoid, occipitalis and masseter. Examination and investigation should be designed to detect other conditions which give rise to headache including cervical spondylosis, ocular or facial sinus diseases, temporomandibular joint disorders and intracranial pathology. Potential treatments include physical, pharmacological and psychological methods. For example, local heat and massage or injection of trigger spots with local anaesthetic may bring a rapid relief. Mild analgesics and short-term administration of minor tranquillisers may also help; diazepam is particularly useful as it not only reduces emotional tension but also relaxes striated muscle. The use of psychological methods, for example, biofeedback and especially relaxation, are helpful in more chronic cases, and counselling or psychotherapy may be needed occasionally.

VASCULAR HEADACHE

Pain arising from blood vessels in the face and head has a throbbing quality unlike the steady ache or stabbing pain of muscle tension. It commonly occurs in generalised disorders giving rise to pyrexia and, in some people, after the consumption of alcohol, after unaccustomed or severe exercise and when in a warm room where ventilation is poor.

MIGRAINE

Known to Hippocrates 2400 years ago and described as 'hemicrania' by Galen in the middle of the 2nd century A.D., this form of headache afflicts about 5 to 10 per cent of adults, being more common in women than men. It tends to appear in adolescence or early adult life and is part of a spectrum of disorders which range from cyclical vomiting and a history of dyspepsia in childhood through true migraine to attacks to vertigo in old age. Often there is a family history of the disorder.

Classical migraine is diagnosed when the sufferer experiences preliminary symptoms, including visual disturbances taking the form of bright flashing lights, difficulties in visual accommodation and sometimes visual field defects which are, fortunately, rarely permanent. These symptoms are related to vaso-constriction of arteries and arterioles in the cranium followed by a period of vaso-dilatation when the headache appears. It is also thought that changes in the size of the venous sinuses of the brain may be involved in the generation of pain. The pain is unilateral (hemicranial), severe and throbbing in nature being associated with photophobia, nausea and, in a severe attack, with vomiting. Pain is mostly experienced in the fronto-temporal region with occipital and sub-occipital pain associated with vertigo, ataxia and vomiting occurring where the basilar artery is primarily involved (basilar migraine). The pain can be extremely severe and although vascular dilatation is cited as its cause hypersensitivity to circulating amines, for example 5-hydroxytryptamine and histamine, both of which are known to be pain producing substances, may well be the chief factor. Hypersensitivity to these substances may also account for the action of ingested amines, for example tyramine in foods which give a food-specific migraine in some sufferers. The most common foods to do this are chocolate (74 per cent), cheese (47 per cent), citrus fruits (32 per cent) and alcohol (25 per cent)—where red wines are the most potent producers of migraine attacks.

Apart from the vascular effects other symptoms indicating hypothalamic disturbances also occur and those recorded include alterations in water balance with increased thirst and water retention before an attack, and diuresis afterwards. Appetite may be increased before the onset of headache, disappearing completely during the attack when anorexia and vomiting occur. There may be an increased desire for sleep. Mood changes with elation or irritation sometimes occur initially with depression and aggression during an attack, occasionally followed by a return of the elated mood afterwards.

In women pre-menstrual migraine is common, suggesting that hormonal changes play some part in the precipitation of attacks. This is supported by the fact that it may begin after the birth of a child, and that 80 per cent of women who suffer from migraine are free from attacks during pregnancy. Oral contraceptives may increase the frequency of attacks or precipitate migraine in those who did not suffer from it previously.

In rare instances a migraine attack leads to neurological sequelae, including paraesthesiae, weakness or paralysis of the contralateral half of the body and perhaps dysphasia or a visual field defect.

Treatment

1. Early in an attack the use of simple analgesics, such as aspirin, may help but administration of an ergotamine preparation is the standard treatment. This may well abort an attack if given at this stage.

2. During an established attack the treatment is symptomatic by means of analgesics and ergotamine preparations, or if the attack is severe by the intramuscular injection of 0.5 mg of ergotamine tartrate. This preparation is also useful where there is pronounced anorexia and vomiting, a situation in which absorption of drugs by the gastro-intestinal route is most unreliable. The patients prefer a darkened room and often like to sleep as the attack comes to a close.

3. Prophylaxis may be achieved by the avoidance of known precipitating factors and also, where attacks are occurring frequently

the use of preparations of ergotamine. However, care should be taken to avoid overdosage of ergotamine and related preparations. Methysergide, which opposes the action of 5-hydroxytryptamine, is sometimes used in prophylaxis but there is a danger that it will cause retroperitoneal fibrosis and its use must be limited to treatment for a maximum period of three months and only where other measures have failed.

VARIANTS OF MIGRAINE

Migrainous neuralgia (cluster headache)
This condition was first differentiated from classical migraine in 1926 by Wilfred Harris, a neurologist. Sufferers from the disorder, which is more common in men than in women and which is familial in 16 per cent of cases, begin to experience bouts of boring, throbbing or burning facial pain in early or middle adult life. It is centred in or around one or other eye and perhaps the cheek or temporal region, occasionally radiating to the shoulder or into the upper teeth of the same side. There is associated photophobia and lacrimation, and sometimes unilateral facial flushing together with blocking of the nostril due to mucosal swelling. The attacks often start in the early morning and may even awaken a person from sleep. The term 'cluster headache' is used because attacks occur frequently for one to three weeks, after which there is a period of freedom which may last six months or more. During a period of headache pain attacks lasting only an hour or so may occur once or more daily and are precipitated by alcohol in particular, though tiredness, over-exertion in sport, lack of food and emotional stress can cause them too. A few patients have daily attacks over many days or even months. The origin of the pain is thought to be similar to that in classical migraine with vascular changes arising as the result of altered activity of the ciliary and sphenopalatine ganglia.

If recognised early cluster headaches respond well to simple analgesics and, in particular, to the administration of ergotamine or an ergot preparation. During a bout of headaches the prophylactic use of drugs described previously for the treatment of the standard form of migraine may be helpful.

POST-TRAUMATIC HEADACHES

After relatively minor head injuries, particularly those sustained during the course of work, or where there is compensation involved, and less so after sport's injuries, persistent headache, together with other symptoms, occurs. Thus, in addition to the headache which is generally located specifically to the point of impact, patients may complain of dizziness, fatigue, irritability, insomnia, nervousness, sensitivity to noise and sometimes of anxiety and depression. In patients with post-traumatic neurosis, the headache often has the characteristics of muscle tension pain. Although some of the symptoms may be physically based upon minor damage to the inner ear, or cervical vertebrae, most are regarded as trivial and therefore if complaints are prolonged, particularly for more than 12 months, they are taken as evidence of an accident neurosis. The reason for post-traumatic headaches is uncertain but there is some evidence that they may be due to a transient increase in the flow of blood through cerebral vessels for a period of weeks after an injury even though it may have been a mild one.

Complaints of persistent headache after severe injuries are, by contrast, relatively uncommon and, if present, short lasting. In both instances the treatment of the pain is by means of simple analgesics and where accident neurosis is thought to be present further investigation by a psychiatrist is advised. Headache may well be due to a specific intracranial lesion and this possibility is described below.

HEADACHE DUE TO RAISED INTRACRANIAL PRESSURE

Intracranial tumour

This is a rare cause of headache and most doctors in general practice will only see one or two cases in their professional lifetime. Pain caused by intracranial tumours is generally due to increased intracranial pressure, either because of the sheer size of the tumour itself, or because it is so placed that, even though small in size, it causes obstruction to the circulation of cerebrospinal fluid through the cerebral ventricles. In some cases pain is due to infiltration of the dura mater by tumour tissue. The pain of raised intracranial pressure is characteristically aching or bursting in nature and felt bilaterally. It is most prominent on waking first thing in the morning often disappearing after an hour or so. It is worsened by coughing, sneezing, bending or straining in any way and, in the later stages, associated with vomiting and mental confusion. Sometimes temporary loss of vision occurs on bending. Examination of the fundus of the eye reveals swelling of the optic nerve head (papilloedema) which, if severe, is associated with retinal haemorrhages. Although not always present a careful examination should be made for signs of focal damage in the central nervous system and a history should be checked for any changes in personality and intellectual function.

Subdural haematoma

An acute subdural haematoma as a result of injury may cause severe focal headache. The history of trauma and evidence of injury, for example local cuts and abrasions or a skull fracture, together with neurological signs and perhaps evidence of rising intracranial pressure indicated by increasing impairment of consciousness, slowing in respiration and rising blood pressure, raises the suspicion of an intracranial abnormality. Surgical investigation and treatment are urgently required. By contrast, a chronic subdural haematoma is associated with a history of trauma in only about half the patients who have one. The latter are most often elderly and the presence of a chronic subdural haematoma should be suspected where there is a history of several days or even weeks of intermittent severe headache and periods of varying consciousness with mental confusion, drowsiness and apathy alternating with clear mental activity. Sometimes evidence of focal neurological damage is present on examination of the central nervous system but this is by no means always the case. Diagnosis is confirmed by skull X-ray (the investigator should search for shifting of the pineal gland from the midline in a postero-anterior view of the skull), angiography or, if available, by computerised axial tomography (brain scan) or isotope brain scan.

Investigation and treatment of serious disorders of brain function causing raised intracranial pressure is a matter for specialist attention by neurologists or neurosurgeons with the onus lying on others to recognise the need for their services.

Subarachnoid haemorrhage

Rupture of an intracranial arterial aneurysm gives rise to sudden and excruciating pain often described as being, 'like a violent blow or kick to the back of the head'. In some cases the sufferer becomes unconscious immediately. Those who do not frequently experience nausea and vomit several times. Pain persists for several days over which it gradually subsides. Nuchal rigidity occurs and its presence together with the pain described is virtually pathognomonic of a ruptured aneurysm. Immediate treatment for pain is by means of oral or parenteral analgesics. The treatment of the cause of the haemorrhage is neurosurgical. Subarachnoid haemorrhage also occurs sometimes in association with head injury giving rise to headache and nuchal rigidity as in the case of a ruptured aneurysm. Similarly, spontaneous cerebral haemorrhage may lead to leakage of blood into the cerebrospinal fluid and give rise to pain.

FACIAL PAIN

Toothache and sinus pain

Toothache due to dental caries is the commonest cause of facial pain. Initially it presents as a complaint by the patient of a vague ache which he or she cannot localise other than to one half of the face. The pain is intermittent and is produced by eating or drinking hot or cold food and fluids, or sweet substances. When the tooth pulp is involved and there is a pulpitis pain is more constant though not necessarily present all the time. The tooth involved can often be located by the patient and by the dentist by percussing the suspected tooth. If a dental abscess forms there is a constant severe local pain and tissue swelling. Occasionally dental pain may be referred to the ear leading to difficulties in diagnosis. After extraction of a tooth, further severe pain may develop about two days later. The condition, known as 'dry socket', is caused by failure of the cavity left by extraction to fill with blood clot, or to dissolution of the clot leaving an empty socket. In addition to pain, the patient has halitosis and swelling of the regional lymph glands. Dental treatment is needed to aid healing of the socket and analgesics should be prescribed.

Sensitivity of the teeth to brushing is often caused by recession of the gingiva from the neck of the tooth leaving the dentine exposed. Inflammation of the gingiva, of which the commonest form is chronic gingivitis, is not painful. The condition is known as pyorrhoea and it gives rise to severe pain only when drainage of an abscess to the gum margin is blocked. The pain is not as severe as an acute pulpitis or periapical inflammation (inflammation around the apex of the root of a tooth).

Pain due to teething occurs in young children and young adults in whom wisdom teeth are erupting. Dull aching pain is experienced around the tooth and in the ear. Generally it lasts for days and may be treated by analgesics if it is severe. Antibiotics may be needed in young adults if infection (pericoronitis) develops in the tissues above the emerging tooth.

Pain due to maxilliary sinusitis gives rise to pain often indistinguishable from toothache, especially where long rooted canines, which lie on the floor of the maxilliary antrum, are covered only by thin bone and mucosa. Here they can be secondarily affected by inflammatory changes within the sinus and an increase in pressure arising as a result of blockage of the outflow of inflammatory products from it. If not located in the canines the pain may well be thought to come from a previously filled tooth, or teeth, which again may mislead the dentist into performing re-explorations. Inflammation in the facial sinuses otherwise gives rise to local pain due to increase pressure as a result of blockage to antral outflow. The affected sinus is located clinically by the site of the pain and the fact that it may be increased by local percussion. There may be redness of the overlying skin and puffiness of the eyes if the tear ducts are blocked. X-ray examination shows loss of translucency of the sinus. It should be remembered that in older patients chronic sinus pain may be due to a tumour.

TRIGEMINAL NEURALGIA

This disorder occurs in middle age and in two thirds of cases after the 50th year affecting women more often than men. Paroxysms of stabbing pain lasting seconds are the characteristic symptom. They are confined to one or perhaps two divisions of the right or left trigeminal nerve, most commonly occurring in the second and third divisions. Pain is triggered by a light touch to the skin of the face, or the mucous membrane, for example during washing, shaving or eating. If it occurs frequently the patient is usually immobilised. Pain seldom disturbs sleep. If symptoms of trigeminal neuralgia occur in a young adult (approximately 1–2 per cent of patients are in this category) the presence of multiple sclerosis should be suspected, although it must be understood that neuralgia is rarely the first sign of this disease. The characteristics of trigeminal neuralgia are:

1. Paroxysms of intense facial pain.
2. Freedom from symptoms between attacks.
3. The presence of trigger sites for pain.
4. The absence of neurological signs of any other kind.

Patients presenting for the first time, irrespective of the origin of neuralgia, should be treated with carbamazepine (Tegretol) in doses of 200 to 600 mg daily, in divided doses. This produces excellent results for two to four years. Alternatively, treatment with phenytoin (Epanutin) in a dose of 200 to 400 mg daily may be helpful. Eventually there is an increasing tendency for the pain to return and when it does surgical treatment involving destruction or division of the appropriate root of the nerve associated with the pain is carried out by a neurosurgeon.

GLOSSOPHARYNGEAL NEURALGIA

This is an uncommon condition similar in nature to trigeminal neuralgia and presenting with bouts of severe stabbing pain deep in the ear and tonsillar region. It is precipitated by swallowing of food and fluids and by coughing or yawning as the trigger zones are the base of the tongue, the pharynx, tonsillar region and the ear. The regime of treatment advised for trigeminal neuralgia should be followed for this condition too.

POST-HERPETIC NEURALGIA

Herpes zoster, or shingles, is most common in later life. It occurs when dormant varicella viruses become active, often many years after invading posterior root ganglia of spinal and cranial sensory nerves. In some way their activity is triggered, often by the presence of other diseases as in the case of malignant disease, or a recent history of irradiation with X-rays. It is most common in the facial region in older women, and in the thoracic region amongst men and the young. In a typical attack of herpes, pain precedes the appearance of a vesicular rash, disappears, and returns after two to three weeks. Post-herpetic pain is severe and burning in nature, at times having a sharp stabbing quality. It is precipitated by light touch, or occurs spontaneously in the region scarred by the vesicular stage of the disease. Though in some patients the pain may disappear gradually over a period of weeks, in others it resists all form of treatment and at times leads to severe depression and even suicide in those who can no longer bear it. The shooting but not the burning pain may be relieved by carbamazepine (Tegretol), but neither are affected by analgesic drugs. Tricyclic antidepressant drugs, such as imipramine, are prescribed at times because they not only promote relief from depression but also seem to have specific analgesic properties too. Pain responds poorly to surgical treatment involving the division or blocking of sensory nerve roots. Recent there have been reports of success in treatment using electrical cutaneous stimulators on the skin of the affected area. However, in the author's experience this form of treatment has only moderate value.

POST-HERPETIC GENICULATE NEURALGIA

This is a specific form of post-herpetic neuralgia where the virus has affected the sensory parts of the facial nerve—the nervus intermedius and geniculate ganglion. As a result the vesicular rash is found on the pinna of the ear and in the external auditory meatus with post-herpetic pain occurring as described above.

ATYPICAL FACIAL PAIN

Pain for which no explanation can be given in terms of an organic lesion sometimes occurs in the distribution of one or other trigeminal nerve, occasionally spreading beyond this to the other side of the face and areas of the neck supplied by upper cervical nerves. It is usually of a dull and aching nature and seems to occur in women of middle age. It is not triggered by cold or touch. The pain may be part of a depressive illness or an hysterical conversion disorder and an attempt should be made to confirm or deny this possibility. Alternatively, the condition may be due to a disturbance of the autonomic supply to facial blood vessels. In patients with this type of pain there will be other signs of disturbed autonomic function, including changes in skin colour and sweat production over the affected part of the face. Treatment is by means of a local anaesthetic block of the stellate or sphenopalatine ganglia.

TEMPOROMANDIBULAR JOINT PAIN

Pain arises as a result of intrinsic joint diseases, such as osteoarthritis or rheumatoid arthritis, and also as a result of disturbances in joint function secondary to malocclusion of the teeth, or to increased clenching of the teeth (Bruxism) in states of emotional stress and chronic tension. In the case of intrinsic joint disease the pain may be unilateral or bilateral and is exacerbated by movements of the jaw. Tenderness of the joint may be elicited by palpation via the external auditory meatus. Abnormalities of the soft tissues around the joint may be evident on inspection and palpation and there may be local tenderness. X-rays of the joint should be carried out to establish whether an arthritic condition is present. The pain of Bruxism is almost always bilateral and examination of the patient will reveal limitation of jaw movement and inability to open the mouth fully as a result of spasm of the masseter muscles, pterygoid muscles and temporalis muscles. On palpation, and in the case of the masseter and pterygoid group this is best done from inside the mouth, tenderness will be felt. However, palpation of the joint through the external auditory meatus does not give rise to pain or tenderness. Treatment for this condition rests upon the solution of the underlying emotional disorder together with the use of simple analgesics and perhaps a muscle relaxant. In cases where joint pathology is present the patient should be referred to a specialist in dental medicine, or a rheumatologist.

ACUTE NECK PAIN

Acute pain in the anterior part of the neck arises where there are inflammatory disorders of the larynx, pharynx and oesophagus and occasionally when pain is referred at the time of a myocardial infarction. In all these disorders the pain will begin suddenly and be surprisingly well localised if arising from structures within the neck. It will be associated with other constitutional disturbances if due to infection or by signs of cardiac abnormalities in the case of an infarct. Acute pain in the posterior cervical muscles occurs in states of raised emotional tension when the pain is located in the suboccipital region. Acute muscle spasm also occurs as the result of minor disturbances in joint function but is rarely due to a cervical disc protrusion or to inflammation of the spinal meninges. In rare cases pain may be due to an intracranial lesion in the posterior fossa of the skull and there is always the possibility that intermittent episodes of pain are due to migraine (see page 64). Patients with inflammation associated with degenerative disorders of the cervical spine, infections of bone or soft tissues and those with lesions in the posterior fossa of the skull complain of muscle stiffness and pain. In addition to local tenderness, which occurs at the site of the disease process or at a distance from it (a muscle trigger spot), limitation of movements of the head and neck also occur.

CHRONIC NECK PAIN

Cervical spondylosis

Cervical spondylosis is the most common cause of chronic pain and limitation of movements of the neck. Degenerative changes in the cervical spine are present in 75 per cent of the population over 50 years of age, but for reasons that are not well understood they produce symptoms in relatively few people.

The process of degeneration centres around the intervertebral fibrocartilaginous discs that separate the vertebrae. With time these shrink and the disc space narrows. As a consequence of a reaction to changes in movement at these joints bony protrusions or osteophytes form on the margins of the vertebrae. In addition, joint ligaments thicken and the spinal canal and foramina through which the nerve roots pass are narrowed. Degenerative changes also occur in the small joints of the vertebrae and if they proceed far enough the combined effects of these changes will be reduction in spinal mobility and pain. The latter is felt locally as a dull ache throughout the posterior cervical region with sharper pains if there is sudden or excessive movement in the joints of the neck. At times more distant pain is felt in the arms as a dull ache which extends from the neck through the trapezius muscles, sometimes reaching the forearms. In addition there may be sharper pains which radiate through the whole length of the arm to the fingers and it is thought that these are due to involvement of cervical nerves which have become compressed or tethered in their dural sheaths as they pass through the spinal foramina. The combination of pain and paraesthesiae in one or both arms forms the basis of the condition of brachial radiculopathy. As degenerative changes are most severe at the interval between the 5th and 6th and between the 6th and 7th vertebrae, these being sites of greatest movement of the spine below the level of the 2nd cervical vertebrae, the pain of nerve involvement is referred to the muscles and dermatomes of the arm and hand (see Fig. 23, p. 180). Nerve compression not only causes pain but also the development of 'pins and needles' or numbness. Muscle wasting is usually slight and changes in reflex activity seldom occurs.

Diagnosis is made on the basis of the history and physical examination with confirmation from X-ray studies of the cervical spine to demonstrate degenerative changes (Table 5). Oblique views of the spine should be obtained in order that the spinal foramina can be examined carefully for occlusion by osteophytes.

Pain tends to wax and wane but treatment will reduce its severity. The basis of treatment is rest, the judicious use of mild analgesics, local heat and gentle massage to reduce muscle spasm. Immobilisation of the cervical spine is also helpful and this can be achieved by the use of a simple home-made collar of foam plastic in a length of tube gauze, or the use of a more sophisticated padded plastic collar made to measure. Greater immobilisation is obtained by bed rest and the use of traction with 5 to 6 lb weights attached to the patient's head by a special harness. Only rarely is surgery indicated and it is performed when there is clear evidence from radiological studies that either nerve root compression by osteophytes or a prolapse of cervical disc material is present and when conservative measures have failed.

Spondylotic headache

Degenerative changes in the cervical spine are a significant cause of headache in individuals in later middle-age and beyond. They complain of persistent dull, nagging pain in the occipital region which is throbbing or lancinating at times and which may radiate to the fronto-temporal region. Pain is precipitated by posture for example,

Table 5 Pain, reflex changes, muscle weakness and sensory changes associated with lesions of cervical nerve roots

Root	Potential pain areas	Muscle weakness	Sensory changes	Reflex changes
C.1	Occiput	Rotation of head		
C.2	Occiput Fronto-temporal	Rotation of head		
C.3	Whole neck, Temporal, posterior facial and sub-mandibular		Parasthesia of cheek and side of neck	
C.4	Whole neck Clavicular and upper scapula areas		Parasthesia along clavicle and upper scapula	
C.5	Deltoid, front of arm to base of thumb	Spinati, deltoid, biceps	Deltoid area	Biceps, Brachioradialis
C.6	Front of arm Radial side hand, thumb and index finger	Biceps, Supinator, Wrist extensors	Thumb and index finger	Biceps
C.6.7 (Commonest)	Outer arm and forearm to index, mid and ring fingers	Triceps and wrist flexors	Index, mid and ring fingers	Triceps
C.8	Inner arm and forearm to mid, ring and little fingers	Ulnar deviation, thumb extensors and adductors	Little finger	

reading, writing, typing or falling asleep in an upright chair. Some sufferers experience greatest pain on waking from a night's sleep. Pain tends to occur in episodes lasting for periods ranging from days to months varying in severity. It is often associated with muscle spasm in the large muscle masses of the neck and shoulders, and trigger points may be present. Head and neck movements are limited. Treatment with simple analgesics and a cervical collar worn especially during sleep, or activities that cause pain, brings a degree of relief to many patients. Injection of trigger points with a local anaesthetic followed by local heat and massage often helps for short periods by reducing muscle spasm.

PAIN IN THE EYE

Pain in the region of the eye may be caused by disease or injury involving the eye or eyelids, or arise from nearby structures in the face and neck or within the skull.

Pain from the eyelids

Infection of the follicle of an eyelash, usually by staphylococci, is known as a stye and is a common and minor cause of pain or, more properly, of discomfort. Treatment by local heat is often all that is required to achieve relief but if the condition recurs several times a local antibiotic cream may be used on the lids and in the anterior nares which act as reservoirs for the bacteria. A small painless cyst of a Meibomian gland produces a hard nodule in the lid known as a chalazion (a hailstone) that can be felt more readily that it can be seen. Infection of a cyst occurs occasionally giving rise to a painful red swelling. If persistent it has to be incised from inside the lid and its contents removed by curettage. An antibiotic cream should be applied locally, and as with other local infections of the lids, a non-systemic form incorporating a mixture of neomycin, polymyxin and bacitracin is used.

Acute infection of a lachrymal gland, dacryocystitis, presents as a painful, red swelling below the inner canthus of the eye. The condition may follow chronic infection with obstruction of the lachrymal duct and watering of the eye as a result of inadequate drainage of tears. Treatment with systemic antibiotics is required, and, if an abscess forms, surgical intervention is needed.

The red, painful eye

Conjunctivitis

Inflammation of the conjunctival mucous membrane is common and may arise as a result of infection with bacteria or viruses, or as an allergic response to topical drug treatments for other disorders of the eye, for example, following the use of atropine drops, penicillin or other antibiotics. Conjunctivitis is caused also by external allergens in the atmosphere, for example pollens in 'hay fever'.

Acute bacterial inflammation is caused commonly by staphylococci or *Diplococcus pneumoniae*. They give rise to hyperaemia (redness), thickening of the conjunctiva, local discomfort rather than pain, often described as 'grittiness', and mild to moderate photophobia. A mucopurulent discharge is produced with the formation of crusts which cause the lids to stick together during sleep. Vision is never impaired and both the cornea and pupil are normal although sometimes infection spreads to give small ulcers at the rim of the cornea. Intra-ocular pressure remains normal. Treatment with non-systemic antibiotic drops every 3 hours in the day and cream at night to prevent the lids sticking gives excellent results in a few days. Care must be taken to distinguish simple conjunctivitis from other causes of conjunctival inflammation, especially corneal ulceration and acute iridocyclitis.

Corneal lesions

Ulceration of the cornea gives rise to moderate to severe pain and the following account is limited to three of the most common causes of this condition, namely, local trauma, bacterial infection and infection by herpes viruses.

The normal cornea is resistant to infection which occurs in most cases only when its surface has been broken by a scratch or foreign body. For example, clumsy removal of a foreign body, using unsterile instruments, or the use of eye drops contaminated by bacteria, will cause ulceration. The symptoms of ulceration are an intense boring pain in and around the eye, watering of the eye and redness of the conjunctiva at the periphery of the cornea nearest to the ulcer. If the ulcer is central the conjunctiva surrounding the entire periphery of the cornea will be reddened. The patient experiences photophobia. Examination of the cornea with a bright light reveals a grey-white and cloudy, non-reflecting area at the site of the ulcer. This is confirmed by staining it green with the vital dye fluorescein.

Infection spreading from the conjunctiva gives rise to a series of small peripherally situated ulcers. A larger central ulcer may be the result of infection with a pneumococcus or other bacteria, and infection with the *Herpes simplex* virus gives rise to a spreading, branching ulcer known as a dendritic ulcer. Bacterial infections are treated with antibiotic drugs but steroids should not be used in this situation or for the treatment of a dendritic ulcer because, although they reduce or abolish redness, they promote extensions of ulceration and this may lead to the serious complication of perforation of the cornea. Idoxuridine is used to treat a dendritic ulcer in the early stages of its formation whereas a chronic or indolent ulcer may have to be carbolised, which means treatment by the application of a small amount of carbolic acid to the surface of the ulcer after anaesthetising the cornea. Patients with dendritic ulcers should be referred to an ophthalmologist for treatment as this is a difficult, potentially dangerous and sometimes lengthy process.

Corneal ulceration occurs as part of the syndrome produced by infection of the ophthalmic division of the trigeminal nerve with the

Herpes zoster virus. Severe pain in the eye is experienced for several days before the rash appears which, if at the tip of the nose, is a sign that the cornea is likely to be involved because both the skin and the cornea are supplied by branches of the nasociliary nerve. By contrast, swelling of the eyelids does not necessarily mean that the cornea is affected. When involved the cornea becomes anaesthetic, oedematous and is covered by many small ulcers caused by rupture of vesicles that form at an early stage in the infection. Inflammation lasts several weeks and usually involves deeper strictures giving rise to an associated iridocyclitis. Treatment by an ophthalmologist is needed and is based upon the use of idoxuridine. Local steroids and atropine are used to relieve pain by reducing inflammation and oedema and by paralysing the iris and ciliary muscle. Systemic analgesics of high potency are required because this disorder gives rise to very severe local pain. Unfortunately the pain may persist for many weeks after signs of infection have disappeared.

Iridocyclitis

The iris, ciliary body and choroid, known collectively as the uveal tract, form a continuous sheet of tissue inside the outer coat of the eye formed by the sclera and cornea. Each element of the tract may become inflamed. If inflammation occurs in the iris and ciliary body the condition is known as iridocyclitis and if confined to the choroid as choroiditis. The former is painful and the latter painless presenting only with impaired vision.

Iridocyclitis causes severe aching pain in and around the eye. It is present even when the lids are closed, it is exacerbated by movements of the eye or local pressure and it wakens patients from sleep. Pain is caused by local oedema and spasm of the iris and ciliary muscles. In addition there is marked photophobia and blepharospasm, or difficulty in opening the eyelids. The eye does not water freely as in conjunctivitis and redness is confined chiefly to the circumference of the cornea; this is known as ciliary injection and is brick-red in colour. Examination reveals that the iris is contracted as a result of spasm and distension with blood. Pus cells accumulate in the anterior chamber of the eye forming a visible collection, or hypopyon, in its lower part under the influence of gravity. Also, the cells adhere to the posterior surface of the cornea and may be visible rather like snowflakes. They are known as keratitic precipitates or K.P. and their presence contributes to blurring of vision. Adhesions may form between the anterior surface of the lens and the iris and are known as posterior synechias.

Pain relief is achieved by use of atropine sulphate drops (1 per cent) two or three times each day with a reduction in the concentration of the solution to 0.5 per cent as the condition improves. This paralyses the iris and ciliary body, and helps to prevent the formation of posterior synechias. Treatment should be carried out with regard for the fact that the use of atropine may precipitate an episode of secondary glaucoma and/or produce a sensitivity reaction involving the eyelids and conjunctiva. Systemic analgesics are usually needed and dark glasses reduce photophobia. Local heat to the eye also aids pain reduction. The inflammation, so long as it is not due to infection, is inhibited by the application of steroid drops or ointment. Iridocyclitis is seldom caused by infection and is mostly self-limiting. Therefore symptomatic relief is the primary aim of treatment and should be administered under the direction of an ophthalmologist. Specific disorders elsewhere in the body associated with this condition include ankylosing spondylitis and Reiter's syndrome.

Acute glaucoma (closed angle glaucoma)
Acute glaucoma almost always occurs in individuals of middle age or older and develops quite suddenly although there may have been warning symptoms for some time beforehand which take the form of intermittent episodes of hazyness of vision, discomfort in the eye and awareness of haloes around bright lights. A major attack begins with the rapid onset of very severe pain in and around the affected eye and with nausea and vomiting. Vision is reduced. Examination reveals dusky congestion around the cornea which appears hazy. Through it the iris can be seen and is dull and green-grey in colour. The pupil is oval, dilated and unresponsive to light. Palpation reveals that the eye is stoney hard and pressure upon it gives rise to increased pain. The symptoms and signs described are caused by a rapid increase in intra-ocular pressure due to obstruction to the normal drainage of aqueous fluid from the anterior chamber of the eye. The condition occurs most often in hypermetropic individuals with a shallow anterior chamber containing a narrow drainage angle.

Treatment, preferably by an ophthalmologist, is needed urgently as vision can be lost in 12 hours from the onset of symptoms. It consists initially of measures designed to reduce intra-ocular pressure and these include the installation of 1 per cent eserine (physostigmine) or 4 per cent pilocarpine drops every few minutes to constrict the pupil and, secondarily, to open the blocked angle of the anterior chamber. Intramuscular acetozolamide (Diamox) in a dose of 250 mg followed by 250 mg oral doses at four hour intervals aids pressure reduction by inhibiting the formation of aqueous fluid. In some cases intravenous urea or mannitol is necessary to achieve this effect. Pain and photophobia are also eased by the use of systemic analgesics, local heat, and an eye pad. After recovery, or after 6 hours if improvement does not occur, surgical treatment involving peripheral iridectomy is carried out. This improves drainage of aqueous fluid permanently and it is usual for the unaffected eye to be treated in the same way to prevent its damage by an acute attack of glaucoma at a later date.

The danger of producing secondary glaucoma with atropine in iridocyclitis has been mentioned and the reader should remember to be careful when considering the use of drugs that have cholinergic effects in the treatment of older patients who might, as a consequence, develop glaucoma. For example, depressed patients above middle age should be given antidepressant drugs with minimal cholinergic effects (see pages 167 and 171–173).

Extra-ocular causes of pain

It is unlikely that the reader will confuse the intrinsic causes of

Table 6 The painful red eye

Symptoms and signs	Acute conjunctivitis	Corneal abrasion, Foreign body, Ulcer	Acute iridocyclitis	Acute glaucoma
Pain	mild discomfort, grittiness	moderate to severe ache	moderate to severe ache	very severe pain
Conjunctival redness	generalised	partially or totally circumcorneal	circumcorneal	circumcorneal
Photophobia	mild	mild to moderate	severe	mild to moderate
Vision	normal	may be impaired	impaired	severely impaired, haloes
Cornea	normal	local ulcer(s) or abrasion	normal ± K.P.	dull and cloudy
Iris/Pupil	normal	normal or small	small, maybe irregular	grey-green, dilated, oval and non-reacting
Tension	normal	normal	may rise due to secondary glaucoma	high, globe very hard and painful on pressure
Discharge	often purulent	watery	watery	slightly watery

ocular pain shown in Table 6 with those arising outside the eye. Migraine, and migrainous neuralgia in particular, are common extra-occular causes of pain and the latter also produces redness of the conjunctiva on the affected side and mild photophobia. Therefore it might be confused with conjunctivitis. Intracranial lesions including certain arterial aneurysms and invasive retro-orbital tumours are uncommon but may present with pain in the region of the eye.

9

Thoracic, abdominal and pelvic pain

Pain in the trunk arises from injury to, or diseases involving one or more of the following structures:

1. Vertebrae, ribs and pelvis.
2. Spinal cord and spinal nerves.
3. Heart, gastro-intestinal tract, biliary tract, pancreas, urogenital tract, pleura and peritoneum.
4. Major blood vessels.
5. Skin and connective tissues.

SKELETAL PAIN

Skeletal pain arises most commonly as a result of trauma or degenerative changes in the bones or joints and invasion by primary or secondary malignant tumours. Infections of bone by tuberculous or pyogenic organisms are not common nowadays although they do occur and developmental anomalies of the spine giving rise to pain are present in the earlier years of life. Many of these conditions can be detected by radiological examination.

General comments upon acute episodic back pain

About 19 million working days are lost annually as a result of back pain in the working population. About 2 million people over the age of 25 years consult their doctor about back pain each year, making this type of disorder one of the commonest seen in general practice. 75 per cent of all concerned are under 65 years of age and half are between 45 and 64 years of age, with women outnumbering men, Chronicity is a common problem and 18 per cent of those who suffer back pain have had their symptoms for more than 20 years, and 20 per cent more than 5 years. Thus there is an enormous pool of individuals who suffer chronic back pain making this one of the most disabling disorders suffered by mankind.

Simple backache is a very common complaint in adult life in both sexes, and approximately 80 per cent of men and 90 per cent of women have had non-specific backache. By contrast children seldom suffer back pains. Pain may be due to one of several causes including the effects of sudden strain due to lifting a heavy weight, a fall, or excessive and unaccustomed physical exercise such as might occur when the amateur gardener takes up his spade with too much enthusiasm in the spring after a winter of contemplation! The cause of backache is seldom determined. It may be due to minor damage to the annular ligament of an intervertebral disc, to joints between the articular facets of adjacent vertebrae, or damage to the fibrous attachments of large muscles of the back to the vertebrae and bones of the sacrum and pelvis. Apart from trivial injuries pain may be related to structural abnormalities of the spine or, much more often, to degenerative changes. Typically, the pain affects overweight manual workers who have experienced trauma, rather than those in sedentary occupations. It is usually a dull ache localised to the lumbar region which limits movement and is associated with local tenderness. It is self-limiting but in the acute stage is relieved by rest, although perhaps not completely abolished by it. When afflicted most people resort to 'home remedies' including the use of local heat, rest and perhaps simple analgesics, with relief in a matter of days. Quite often problems of this kind, if they persist, are taken to an osteopath, especially by athletes, and most do not reach a doctor. Medical help is generally sought by those of an over-anxious nature, those who need a certificate for a day or two from work, and those who have prolonged suffering which does not resolve in response to simple remedies. Though many cases of simple backache are due to stress, bad posture, obesity, excessive exercise or any combination of these, the doctor should be alert to the fact that backache may well herald the presence of disease of the spine, the pelvic organs, upper gastro-intestinal tract and pancreas. It is often a presenting symptom of major disturbances of emotional life too: in fact about one third of those with simple backache who appear in their general practitioner's surgery have emotional problems, although the two are not always directly related.

In adolescents and young adults complaints of persistent backache may be due to congenital anomalies of the spine, or to the onset of a rare condition, ankylosing spondylitis. Later in life, and in the middle years, degenerative changes give rise to back pain quite often the most specific form being due prolapse of a lumbar intervertebral disc. Disc prolapse in the thoracic spine is, by contrast, a very rare occurrence. In middle life sacro-iliac strain with local pain is quite common, especially amongst women, and at this time pain due to malignant disease begins to appear, usually as a result of a secondary spread from a carcinoma of the lung, breast or stomach, and in later life amongst men from the prostate gland. Occasionally a primary malignant tumour develops and causes pain. Usually it is a single myeloma or part of the disorder of multiple myelomatosis. Amongst women backache frequently occurs as a normal feature of menstruation and pregnancy and at any time of life as a symptom of disease in the pelvic organs. Finally, osteoporosis is a cause of back pain in the elderly and in some patients this reaches very severe levels.

Myofascial trigger points

A trigger point in a skeletal muscle, so named because pressure upon it 'fires off' pain, is a thickened band of muscle fibres commonly located at the junction of the muscle and its tendon or along one of its borders. Trigger points are not present in a normal muscle and appear only after damage to it has been caused by local disease or injury, or an abnormality in a nearby joint. For example, they develop after sports' injuries, domestic injuries, injuries at work, following surgical operations and, on occasions, in association with visceral diseases. The condition of 'lumbago', described in the next section, is an example of a myofascial syndrome. Trigger points give rise to local tenderness and a deeper, more diffuse aching pain. They are easily detected by drawing the forefinger firmly across the painful area in several directions. Pressure upon the point increases pain and may give rise to referred pain at a distance from the point. Each muscle group has a specific area to which pain is referred. This is not a widely recognised phenomenon and accounts for a substantial number of unexplained cases of chronic pain in all parts of the body. Apart from local pressure, passive stretching of the affected muscle gives rise to pain as does its use in active resistance of movement; a manoeuvre known as isometric contraction. Weakness and restriction of movement occur in association with pain and it has been reported that abnormal vasomotor and other autonomic changes occur in the area of referred, diffuse, deep tenderness. These include vasoconstriction, pallor, sweating and coldness of the skin which are reversed by abolition of the trigger point by injection.

Treatment of myofascial pain has gone through many changes and current practice consists of three stages. First, the trigger point is located and then pain is eliminated either by infiltration with a local anaesthetic or by using the 'dry needling' technique of acupuncture although this produces an increase in pain initially. Pain relief is also produced by sudden, intense cooling of the skin overlying the point with an ethyl chloride spray. Having abolished local tenderness the muscle is very gently and passively stretched thus avoiding further injury whilst stretching the intense local contraction at the site of the trigger point. Finally, the patient is encouraged to use the muscle actively but with only a light work load at first. It seems that once established trigger points are likely to recur at intervals in response to further local injury or, in some cases, in response to heightened emotional tension. Thus, in patients who exhibit emotional tension and have one or more trigger points the effectiveness of treatment will be enhanced by the use of a more general relaxation technique in addition to the measures described. Small doses (5 mg) of diazepam also help to relieve tension.

Lumbago

This term is used to describe acute attacks of low transverse backache brought about by excessive strain in the area and it is probably caused by some tearing of lumbar muscle fibres or of their attachments to bone and associated secondary muscle spasm. The latter can be felt on palpation and careful examination of the area will reveal acutely painful nodules. The pain is very severe at times and, with it, there will be loss of movement of the lumbar spine which becomes stiff or even rigid. However, there will be no evidence of nerve root involvement on examination of muscle power, sensation and reflexes of the lower limbs, and radiological investigations mostly reveal a normal spine. Treatment is by rest, the use of simple analgesics and local heat by means of hot water bottles or, if available, in infra-red lamp. The condition generally clears within a matter of days. In more severe cases infiltration of local anaesthetic into 'trigger spots' may hasten relief as may the use of muscle relaxant drugs, where those with a central action on the nervous system, for example diazepam, have the added advantage of reducing the emotional tension that often accompanies acute pain.

Sacro-iliac pain

Strain or tearing of some fibres of the ligaments binding the sacro-iliac and lumbo-sacral joints gives rise to a low generalised backache with acute pain on pressure over the joints involved. It occurs in association with unaccustomed exercise or exertion and seems to be more common amongst women. In an acute form this disorder arises during later pregnancy or after parturition in a small number of women secondary to excessive relaxation of all ligaments of the pelvic joints due to circulation of an unidentified endogenous substance, called 'relaxin'. Sacro-iliac strain, as with other muscular and ligamentous causes of simple backache, is frequently associated with obesity, and weight reduction, together with rest, local heat and analgesics, are usually sufficient to terminate an attack and reduce the chances of further episodes. Where excessive relaxation of pelvic ligaments occurs the patient should be given a corset or even be wrapped firmly in a roller towel whilst being kept in bed to relieve both pain and reduce the uncomfortable sensation that the pelvis is 'falling apart'. The condition usually settles within a matter of a week or so.

Ankylosing spondylitis

This is a rare condition, the cause of which is unknown. It afflicts men rather more than women and although rare in its full form it is thought to occur in a minor way in 1 to 1.5 per cent of the adult population. It appears in the early years of adult life. Its cause is unknown and initially patients present with complaints of low backache which is most obvious in the morning when there is also marked stiffness. With time the disease process, which first involves the sacro-iliac joints, takes in other joints as it ascends the spine to give a 'bamboo spine', so called because of its appearance on radiographs. The degree of progression is variable — in some it halts when disability is quite mild, but in others it may progress until the whole spine is involved and becomes completely ossified leaving the individual bent like a bow and unable to see ahead because of the extreme degree of fixed spinal flexion. Diagnosis usually rests upon the history and the presence of sclerosis in the joints on a radiograph, especially the sacroiliac joints, although there may not be evidence of such changes for a year or more after the onset of pain. A radioscintiscan is more useful than an X-ray in detecting early stages of sacro-ilitis, and the presence of a raised erythrocyte sedimentation rate is significant in diagnosis. Treatment is by means of analgesics and the use of steroid drugs.

Prolapsed invertebral disc

Prolapse of intervertebral disc material in the lumbar region is far more common than in the thoracic spine, though both are amongst the less common causes of back pain. In fact, approximately 8 per cent of men and 6 per cent of women who complain of back pain to their family doctor have lumbar disc disorders. Of these two-thirds will be attending with a first attack of pain and will have had symptoms for less than two weeks. Most protrusions are from the discs between the 5th lumbar and 1st sacral vertebrae and the 4th and 5th lumbar vertebrae, the former being affected about twice as often as the later. Involvement of lumbar discs at a higher level

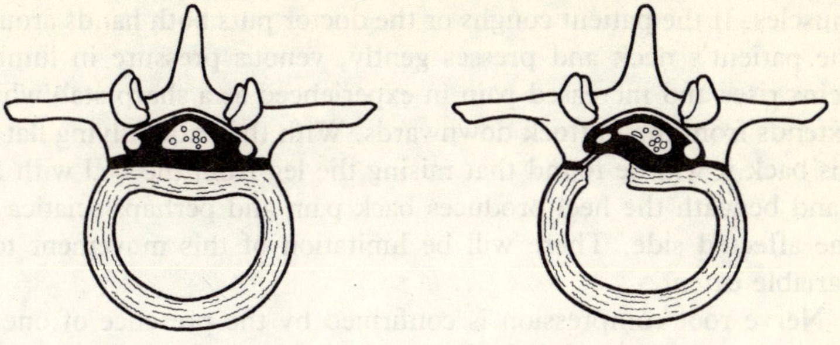

Fig 21. A lateral lumbar disc protrusion (from Jennett, W.B. 1964)

occurs much less frequently. The symptoms include low backache and leg pain (sciatica) if disc material protrudes and compresses a nerve root. The protrusion is usually lateral though occasionally central (Fig. 21). An episode of backache and sciatica is in many cases preceded by a history of one or more attacks of lumbago or lumbar pain over a period of months or years. Men in their thirties and forties are most often afflicted and, although a prolapse may be due to an episode of unaccustomed exercise, an awkward twist of the back, or the lifting of an unusually heavy weight, this is not necessarily so in every case. The attack may be rapid in onset with simultaneous appearance of back pain and sciatica but often back pain precedes the sciatica by a matter of several hours or even a day or two. When it appears the sciatic pain radiates first into the buttock and then through the posterior thigh reaching the calf and possibly the lateral aspect of the foot.

The first pains experienced are probably caused by a rupture of fibres of the degenerate fibro-cartilaginous annular ligament which encloses the softer central core or nucleus pulposus of the disc. Sciatica occurs when disc material protrudes backwards through a rupture in this ligament to compress a nerve root or roots.

The pain is not constant in severity as it is worsened by coughing, sneezing, straining at the time of defaecation, or by bending. Many patients complain of not being able to sit comfortably and prefer to stand or lie down because in this way they prevent increased tension on the trapped nerve roots by avoiding flexion of the lumbar spine.

On examination there is usually a limp and often a scoliosis to right or left. The degree of lumbar lordosis, or antero-posterior curvature, which is normally present in the lumbar area is lost, the lumbar muscles are usually in spasm and this is most obvious on the side of the scoliosis. On examination there is local tenderness in the muscles. If the patient coughs or the doctor puts both hands around the patient's neck and presses gently, venous pressure in lumbar veins rises and increased pain in experienced as a sharp stab which extends from the buttock downwards. With the patient lying flat on his back it will be found that raising the leg from the bed with the hand beneath the heel produces back pain and perhaps sciatica on the affected side. There will be limitation of this movement to a variable extent.

Nerve root compression is confirmed by the presence of one or more signs indicating their dysfunction. These are the presence of numbness or 'pins and needles' in the dermatome supplied by the nerve(s) and, reduction or absence of tendon reflexes, diminution or loss of sensation to touch or pin-prick, and weakness of appropriate muscles (see Table 7 and Fig. 22). On the rare occasions when a central disc protrusion has occurred signs and symptoms are bilateral and if compression of the cauda equina is present there will be abnormalities of bladder and anal sphincter function with urinary retention and constipation. Most patients are relieved by simply resting in bed and symptomatic treatment with analgesics. The bed should be level and firm and can be stiffened by placing boards beneath the mattress. Patients must lie completely flat with one pillow only and remain in bed for a period of one to three weeks, depending upon the severity of the attack and the rate of recovery. This constraint will ensure that excessive spinal flexion is avoided. After a period of bed rest patients are allowed to get up for increasing periods of time, but advised that when sitting they should choose

Table 7 Neurological signs produced by compression of lumbar and sacral nerve roots by prolapsed intravertebral disc material

Nerve root	Vertebral level	Pain and sensory loss	Motor weakness	Reflex changes
L.3	L.2/3	Front of lower thigh	Extension of knee	Knee jerk reduced or absent
L.4	L.3/4	Medial calf and lower leg	Extension of knee. Dorsiflexion of foot	Knee jerk reduced or absent
L.5	L.4/5	Lateral calf and lower leg. Dorsum of foot	Dorsiflexion of foot	No reflex change
S.1	L.5/S1.	Lateral border foot. Sole of foot and lower back of leg	Plantar flexion of foot	Ankle jerk reduced or absent

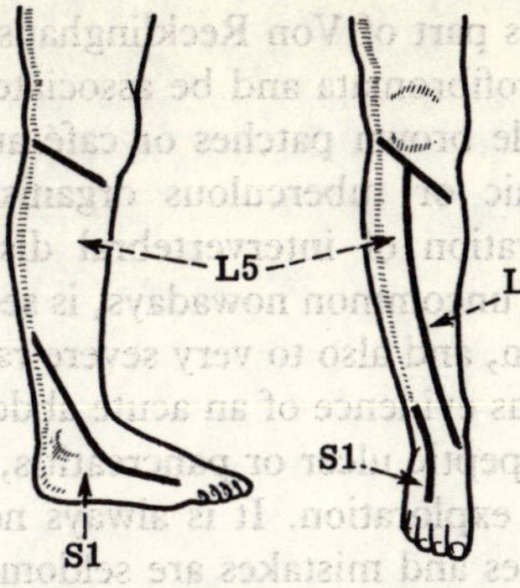

Fig 22. Dermatomes of the lower limb

a firm chair with a straight back in order to avoid excessive spinal flexion. A lumbar support or surgical corset is not ordinarily recommended, though opinions vary about this, and physiotherapy with back extension exercises is regarded as being of value because it restores lost lumbar muscle power and tone, thereby protecting the lumbar spine from excessive and abnormal movements. When an attack is not relieved by these simple measures and pain, with or without neurological signs, persists, the advice of an orthopaedic surgeon or neurosurgeon is advised as specialist treatment may be required. This may mean the use of skin traction, greater immobilisation by means of a fabric, steel or plaster jacket, and perhaps surgery for the removal of the prolapsed intervertebral disc material if there are signs of nerve root compression. Of those in Britain who undergo surgical treatment about 80 per cent will remain free from further signs and symptoms, 10 per cent will develop further pain and sciatica that will be relieved by surgery, and 10 per cent are likely to suffer from chronic pain in the lumbar region, perhaps accompanied by pain radiating into the leg.

Pain from spinal disorders

Diseases or degenerative conditions, primarily or secondarily involving the spinal cord and nerve roots, at times give rise to pain in the chest, abdomen, pelvis or lower limbs. Diseases of the thoracic segments of the cord, of which the most common is multiple sclerosis, may give rise to pain which radiates from the dorsal region along the lines of distribution of the 3rd to the 10th thoracic nerves in the chest and abdomen. For example, a simple neurofibroma of a dorsal nerve root, which is the commonest primary tumour in this part of the nervous system, will give rise to severe back pain and increased sensitivity to touch and pinprick in the distribution of the appropriate nerve. As part of Von Recklinghausen's disease it may be one of many neurofibromata and be associated with the characteristic cutaneous pale brown patches or café au lait spots. Spinal infection by pyogenic or tuberculous organisms with vertebral collapse or disintegration of intervertebral discs and nerve root compression, though uncommon nowadays, is seen occasionally and gives rise to local pain, and also to very severe radiating pain which is at times mistaken as evidence of an acute abdominal catastrophe, such as a perforated peptic ulcer or pancreatitis, thereby leading to unnecessary surgical exploration. It is always necessary to bear in mind such possibilities and mistakes are seldom made in diagnosis if clinical histories are carefully elicited accompanied by appropriate radiological investigations where suspicion is aroused that abdominal or chest pain may be due to disease in the spine.

Backache and emotion

There are two ways in which emotion is associated with back pain and attention must be given to this relationship when planning treatment. First, anxiety, hysterical and hypochondriacal personality traits, may lead to varying degrees of magnification of, or to excessive and persistent preoccupation with, pain which has an organic cause. Second, in the absence of organic disease, psychological factors may lead to the development of low back pain and both these possibilities are described in detail elsewhere (see pages 46–48 and 130–133). It is often stated that pain strongly related to emotional but not to organic factors can only be diagnosed by exclusion of physical causes but attention to both physical and emotional components of a clinical problem show that this is not so and that the diagnosis of pain can be made without resorting to laboratory tests other than simple radiology and perhaps an erythrocyte sedimentation rate. For example, several groups of signs may be detected during physical examination which favour a psychological bias in the patient's presentation. The signs, which are described below, are most reliable in patients under 50 years of age.

1. Over-reaction to examination with exaggerated facial expressions, movements, and complaints of pain, with sweating and/or 'collapsing' during the procedure.

2. Increased sensitivity to light pinching of the skin over a wide area of the back and complaints that deep pressure causes widespread tenderness.

3. Inappropriate reports of pain when rotational movement of the spine is simulated by rotating the patient's shoulders and pelvis in

the same plane; a manoeuvre that does not rotate the spine but to the patient seems to do so.

4. Downward pressure on the spine through the shoulders, or axial loading, produces complaints of pain although this rarely happens when a spinal disorder is present.

5. Normal clinical examination reveals marked impairment of straight-leg raising with the patient lying down but when asked to sit up on the examination couch he or she manages to do so without pain despite the fact that the legs are flexed to 90°. Distraction of the patient by engaging him or her in conversation tends to increase the sensitivity of this test.

6. Examination of muscle groups may reveal jerky 'giving way' of the muscles without any relation to specific myotomes and inappropriate sensory changes, for example, diminished sensation which does not match accepted dermatome distributions (see Fig. 23).

Caution is advised in the use of the signs described because none of them in itself is sufficient to enable the clinician to conclude that psychological factors are the primary cause of pain. There should be at least three signs present before this conclusion is reached. For further information the reader is advised to consult a paper by Waddell and others entitled 'Non-organic physical signs in low-back pain' (Spine, 5, 117–125, 1980).

NON-SKELETAL THORACIC PAIN

Thoracic pain may arise from the viscera; the heart and the oesophgus, from the parietal pleura but not the visceral pleura, in addition to chest wall structures including the skin, ribs and muscles.

Cardiac pain

The heart has always played a central hole in man's emotional life and it is therefore not surprising that anxiety about its dysfunction is common. Such anxieties are at times associated with chest pains and must be distinguished from pain arising as a result of ischaemia of heart muscle. The latter is most often felt retrosternally and through the chest wall in the distribution of the first five thoracic nerves because they are involved in the sympathetic nerve supply to the heart. As sympathetic inflow occurs at the first thoracic level, pain may also be experienced in the distribution of nerves to the left arm with radiation as far as the thumb. Because of the connection of the sympathetic nerve supply of the head and neck with the upper thoracic segments of the cord into which it flows, pain may also be felt along the left side of the neck, in the jaw and, at times, over the face. Classically, ischaemic pain is severe and aching in nature encircling the chest and becoming a crushing sensation if the product of a myocardial infarct.

The pain of angina pectoris occurs where temporary ischaemia has been produced by imposing too great a work load on the heart. This may occur during walking, or climbing stairs, or as a result of heightened emotion. The pain disappears quickly when the load lessens or the sufferer uses a drug, such as glyceryl trinitrate, to dilate the coronary arteries. In addition to dilating the coronary arteries this drug also causes more general vascular dilatation and thereby reduces the work of the heart. The pain of a myocardial infarction, on the other hand, is persistent, unrelieved by rest and not necessarily related to a period of exercise or exertion. When severe it is associated with signs of circulatory collapse, the patient being ashen in colour and having a clammy skin and low blood pressure. Such an episode is also accompanied by considerable anxiety and apprehension. An infarct does not always produce severe pain for, on occasions, the symptoms may be so mild as to be regarded as due to indigestion.

Chest pain related to emotional stress

Complaints of aching pain confined to the left side of the chest, especially in the nipple area and below and apparently linked with exercise, should be viewed with considerable suspicion especially if unaccompanied by any form of electrocardiographical evidence of heart disease. In the patient's mind the pain may not be associated with an emotional cause and therefore it arouses considerable anxiety. As he or she believes it is due to heart damage it may well be accompanied by pallor, sweating and panic, as in those who have myocardial disease. Because of its positive association with exercise the disorder is sometimes known as the effort syndrome or a cardiac neurosis. Physical investigations are negative, but psychological enquiries may well reveal evidence of chronic or acute anxiety, hypochondriasis or hysterical elements in the personality. The pain may arise acutely in states of sudden stress, for example amongst soldiers in battle or after the loss of a relative or friend from heart disease, especially if death occurred as a result of myocardial infarction.

Epidemic myalgia (Bornholm's disease)

This condition is due to viral infection and gives rise to chest pain which is acute in onset and severe. Generally the pain is unilateral and may be mistaken for pain of myocardial infarction. If there is doubt the patient should be subjected to the usual laboratory tests for disturbances of enzyme function and an electrocardiogram. A search should be made for evidence of associated pericarditis, orchitis and encephalitis.

Pleuritic pain

Pain from the parietal, mediastinal and diaphragmatic areas of the pleura is severe, stabbing in nature and fluctuates with respiratory movements. It is sharpest on inspiration and attempts to minimise it lead to shallow and short breaths. Parietal pleuritic pain is experienced in the chest wall and occurs chiefly in association with underlying acute bacterial infections of the lung. It may also occur when there is infiltration by tumour, for example from the breast or lung, or more rarely where the tumour arises from the pleura itself as in the case of a mesothelioma. Pain due to irritation of the mediastinal pleura in an infectious disorder of the lung or mediastinal contents is experienced retrosternally, in the neck, and the shoulders. The pleura over the central area of the diaphragm is supplied by the 3rd, 4th and 5th cervical segments of the spinal cord through the phrenic nerve and pain arising from it is experienced as referred pain over the shoulder tip. This may happen in basal pneumonia or where there is an acute inflammation of the gallbladder affecting the under surface of the diaphragm. The outer third of the diaphragmatic pleura is supplied by the intercostal nerves and any pain arising from it will be experienced over the chest wall.

Spontaneous pneumothorax

This disorder is characterised by the sudden onset of moderate to severe pain localised to the lateral or anterior chest wall. It is aggravated by coughing and associated with breathlessness. Apart from spontaneous rupture of a bulla on the surface of the lung, the condition may be caused by piercing of the lung by the bone spicules from fractured ribs. The history and clinical examination are usually sufficient to make the diagnosis, and chest X-ray should be performed to confirm it.

Oesophageal pain

Pain arising from the oesophagus is surprisingly well localised to the neck or chest. It is felt either as a discomfort or burning pain, or as an acute local pain worsened by swallowing. Localisation may be aided by the fact that disorders of the upper oesophagus give rise to a sensation sensation of a projection within its lumen. In the condition of hiatus hernia where pain arises from the lower oesophagus due to reflex of stomach contents it is felt in the chest and retrosternally and may be confused with pain due to a peptic ulcer.

Herpes zoster

The dorsal root ganglia of the thoracic nerves are commonly involved in infection by herpes zoster virus. The clinical features have been described earlier (see page 71) and as in the case of facial herpes, post-herpetic neuralgia is a serious complication amongst older people. Patients soon learn that their pain can be reduced by firm pressure over the affected area and at times arrive for clinical examination wearing either a silk or other smooth garment next to the skin, perhaps having bound their chest wall firmly, first placing a piece of fine material over the painful area. Treatment of the condition is also described on page 71.

NON-SKELETAL ABDOMINAL PAIN

Abdominal pain arises from a variety of causes, the most common of which are shown in Table 8.

Table 8 Common causes of abdominal pain

Viscera involved	Cause of pain
Stomach and duodenum	Hiatus hernia
	Gastric ulcer
	Duodenal ulcer
Small and large bowel	Intestinal obstruction
	(e.g. by tumour; bowel herniation, 'adhesions')
	Ulcerative colitis
	Appendicitis
	Diverticulitis
Biliary tract	Cholecystitis
	Biliary colic
Pancreas	Acute and chronic pancreatitis
Renal tract	Acute and chronic pyelonephritis
	Renal colic
	Cystitis
	Retention of urine
Female reproductive organs	Dysmenorrhoea
	Ectopic pregnancy
Infection	Chemical and bacterial peritonitis

Peptic ulcer pain

Peptic ulceration is included amongst those disorders which are regarded as psychosomatic (see pages 129, 130). Of the two forms of peptic ulceration that occur, namely gastric and duodenal, it is the latter which predominates being most common amongst men and amongst those of blood group 'O'. Thus there is undoubtedly an hereditary factor involved in the development of a duodenal ulcer and predisposition to it probably leads to ulcer formation and pain, when emotional and environmental circumstances are appropriate. In other words, the onset of symptoms is due to the effect of several different but important factors acting in unison. The symptoms of the disorder vary in intensity and disappear at times, occasionally for months or even years. There is a significant relationship between their appearance, severity, and personal stress, but this is not always the case. A significant relation between any particular personality characteristic and a tendency to ulcer formation has not been proved although it is often said that tense, driving and over-ambitious individuals are more susceptible than most.

The chief symptom of peptic ulceration is well localised epigastric gnawing discomfort which is only rarely regarded by the patients as a truly painful experience. In some cases, patients waken in the morning with nausea and may retch or occasionally vomit bile-stained fluid. Discomfort or pain arises from the ulcer base which is exposed to gastric contents. If an ulcer is on the posterior wall of the stomach or first part of the duodenum, it may give rise to pain both in the epigastrium and in the back just below the left scapula. The pain is caused by hydrochloric acid which breaches the protective layer of mucin which normally lines the gastrointestinal tract. The pains of gastric and duodenal ulceration are said to be distinguishable from the patient's history by the fact that gastric symptoms tend to occur within an hour or so of meals, whereas duodenal pain will not appear for one to four hours. In many cases this turns out to be speculative and confirmation is obtained from a barium meal and perhaps from endoscopy. When an ulcer perforates, and such an episode is not always preceded by an obvious history of peptic ulceration, the gastric contents come into contact with the peritoneum and initially give rise to chemical peritonitis which, if untreated, becomes a bacterial one. Pain associated with perforation is usually very severe, local at first, and then more generalised as peritoneal soiling spreads. In response to inflammation the muscles of the abdominal wall become rigid or board-like and attempts to palpate lead to further pain. The patient has a pallid, cold and clammy skin and a dramatic fall in blood pressure as part of the process of haemodynamic shock. If the perforation is a small one and the contents leak only slowly into the abdominal cavity, trickling down the lateral side of the ascending colon, the pattern of pain may closely resemble that of an inflamed appendix and be mistaken for it.

In most cases of peptic ulceration treatment is by means of judicious dietary restrictions, that is leaving out from the diet those foods known to cause discomfort or pain, the use of alkalis such as magnesium hydroxide to relieve symptoms, or, in persistent and resistant cases, bed rest, antacids and diet, antispasmodics, or the drug Tagamet (cimetidine) in a dose of 200 ml three times daily with meals and 400 ml at night. Healing of the ulcer takes place in 85 per cent of patients treated and acid production is reduced in 70 per cent. When acute symptoms have subsided, a maintenance dose of Tagamet of 400 ml at night may be required. On cessation of treatment, the risk of recurrence returns to the pre-treatment level. Ranitidine (Zantac) is a newer drug of the same type and has similar properties and side-effects other than the production of gynaecomastia when used for long periods. It is given in doses of 150 mg twice daily to a maximum of 900 mg daily in divided doses. The maintenence dose is 150 mg at bedtime. Where necessary psychological methods are used either in the form of drug therapy with minor tranquillisers at times of emotional stress, or simple discussions with the patient designed to ameliorate or remove stressful influences in the home or elsewhere. Various forms of surgery are available and are usually resorted to only when all medical forms of treatment have proved unsatisfactory, and the indications for this kind of therapy is a matter for specialist opinion. However whatever form of surgery is carried out, the individual who is least likely to benefit will show evidence of poor emotional resources when exposed to stress and/or a family and social environment which gives relatively little support. The converse is true in general for the emotionally well-balanced individual and for those who come from a supportive social and emotional background.

Carcinoma of the stomach

This disease causes marked weight loss, profound or absolute anorexia, anaemia and, in some cases, discomfort or pain which is of an aching or gnawing nature perhaps radiating to the back. In some patients it takes the form of a colic. Pain and discomfort may be relieved by food or, alternatively, by vomiting. The volume of vomit is often large, it contains food taken some time previously and perhaps fresh or altered blood which gives it a brownish colour. Diagnosis is made by means of a good history and examination for an epigastric mass produced by the tumour or the stomach distended with fluid. Confirmation is by means of endoscopy and/or radiography.

Ulcerative colitis

This disease occurs chiefly in early adult life. It is a familial disorder which was first described in 1875 and it is one of the classical psychosomatic disorders, (see page 129). It is characterised clinically by bouts of lower abdominal pain which varies from mild to severe cramps, anorexia, nausea, and frequent loose stools. The main constituents of the latter are blood and mucus. The more proximally the disease extends in the colon the more likely it is that the stools will be loose and unformed. In association with spontaneous pain palpation of the abdomen reveals generalised tenderness. The condition is associated in some cases with arthritis and other systemic manifestations, including systemic lupus erythematosus. Its origins are subject to considerable debate and, apart from speculation about the role of genetic factors, infectious causes and allergies, emotion has long been regarded as significant in the precipitation or worsening of attacks of the disease. It is clear, as with peptic ulceration, that a genetic predisposition and the individual's emotional constitution are important, with the latter being involved in both the precipitation of attacks and methods of coping with symptoms. Studies of the interrelation between physical and psychological symptoms have failed to reveal a susceptible personality type but show that emotionally significant events, whether pleasant or unpleasant, may trigger attacks of pain and bloody stools in susceptible individuals. It has also been shown that those from unstable or emotionally poor environments are at significant risk given that they are constitutionally susceptible to the disease. The disease itself often gives rise to considerable anxiety or depression reflecting the degree to which it threatens the patient's emotional, social and financial stability.

As implied, ulcerative colitis is a phasic disorder of varying degrees of severity. Medical control with drugs, such as Salazopyrin (0.5 g four times daily for mild attacks and maintenance, and 1 g four times daily for acute episodes) and the use of a low roughage diet, iron supplements for anaemia and relief from stress, if necessary supported by psychotherapy, is often sufficient to maintain reasonably good health. Steroids are used in the treatment of more severe cases. Prednisolone in a dose of 5 mg four times daily is prescribed in addition to Salazopyrin and, if the symptoms are more severe, this may rise to 40 to 60 mg per day given in association with steroid enemas, as many as two to three times daily, until control is gained. The reader should consult more specialised texts for the full details of treatment programmes for this disease. Surgery, entailing total colectomy with the fashioning of an ileostomy, is recommended when the disorder is chronic with unremitting diarrhoea, bleeding, malaise and chronic sepsis. Usually it is elective but, in a fulminating attack where perforation of the bowel threatens, surgery is required as an emergency procedure.

Obstruction and inflammation

Pain due to obstruction of a viscus, its duct, or a segment of bowel, if sudden in onset, is acute but intermittent. Irrespective of the organ involved the pain is called a 'colic', meaning that its pattern is rhythmical with peaks at times of muscle contraction and distension. There is complete relief or a dull background ache in the interludes between episodes of colic.

Biliary colic

This is caused by obstruction and distension of the hepatic ducts or more often of the common bile duct by calculi (gallstones) formed in the gallbladder. Colic is localised to the right hypochondrium and dull back pain also occurs in the region of the right scapula over the distribution of the sixth to the eighth thoracic nerves which receive sensory afferent nerve fibres from the gallbladder. Shoulder tip pain also occurs where the gallbladder has afferent connections via the phrenic nerve with the third, fourth and fifth cervical segments of the spinal cord, or where the pleura of the central area of the diaphragm becomes inflamed. Small calculi may ultimately pass into the duodenum but larger ones can cause prolonged obstruction damming back bile producing a clinical picture of obstructive jaundice.

When colic is present symptomic relief is gained by intramuscular injections of pethidine. Morphine is not used as it causes closure of the sphincter of the common bile duct. Surgery entails removal of the obstruction and usually the gallbladder also which is the site of formation of calculi.

Renal colic

Renal colic is a very severe pain caused by the passage of a renal calculus down the ureter from the renal pelvis. It may traverse the length of the ureter to reach the bladder or cause permanent obstruction of the ureter with dilatation of the renal pelvis hydronephrosis and failure of kidney function eventually. The nerve supply of the renal pelvis and ureter consists of autonomic plexuses in their walls originating from the renal and hypogastric plexuses. Many of the nerve fibres in them are concerned with sensation and afferent nerves pass to the eleventh and twelfth thoracic and to the first lumbar segments of the cord. Pain, which is most probably due to a rapid rise in intra-luminal pressure in the renal pelvis and ureter, is therefore experienced at first in the loin on the affected side and then, as the calculus passes towards the bladder, in the flank and inguinal region. It may radiate to the testis in the male, the labium majus in the female and anterior aspect of the thigh in both. Apart from the passage of a calculus, renal colic is produced by blood clot, polyps and spasm of the ureter without the presence of an obstructing intra-luminal body. Less than half all patients with colic have a calculus or other intra-luminal mass. Inflammation of the renal pelvis in pyelonephritis, which may occur in association with hydronephrosis, gives rise to a more steady but severe loin pain together with general features of an infection, namely malaise, fever, anorexia and perhaps headache.

The immediate treatment of renal colic is by means of intramuscular pethidine or in severe cases by intravenous administration of this drug. If the block perists surgery is required.

Bladder calculi are uncommon nowadays except in patients who have been catheterised or bedridden for many months especially if there has been recurrent infection. In well-managed patients such complications are minimal but nevertheless do occur. Pain when present occurs if the patient is sitting or standing, because the stone irritates the trigone area. Its severity is increased by riding in a jolting vehicle and towards the end of micturition when, in men, it radiates to the tip of the penis and may be associated with the passage of free blood or blood clots in the urine. Pain due to inflammation of the bladder, for example in cystitis, is described as a diffuse low abdominal ache which changes to a burning sensation at the time of micturition. It is associated with low back pain. The passage of small calculi through the urethra gives rise to acute local pain, persistent soreness for some hours afterwards and quite often there is a small amount of blood passed with the calculus.

The treatment of bladder infections entails the use of antibiotic or antimicrobial drugs to which the infecting organisms are sensitive. The patients are encouraged to drink freely, thus flushing the bladder, and an intake of about two litres a day is sufficient for this purpose. Bladder calculi of a small size are often passed through the urethra, but larger ones may have to be crushed in situ and the debris washed from the bladder. The other chief cause of bladder pain is malignant disease which may be primary or arise in organs nearby.

Peritoneal pain

Pain due to chemical or bacterial irritation of the peritoneum is acute and well localised if it involves the parietal layer and is duller and more diffuse if it originates in the visceral layer. The difference between the nature and localisation of the two is well illustrated by considering the sequence of events that occurs during an attack of appendicitis leading to the rupture of this part of the bowel. A similar sequence of events may also be observed in diverticulitis of the colon. In this case the pain is located to the left of the abdomen rather than to the right. Infection of the appendix is associated with obstruction in the normal outflow of its contents, and as a result the early stages of the disorder may produce a mild abdominal colic. Inflammation confined to the appendix and its peritoneum leads to increased activity of autonomic afferent nerves which enter the tenth, eleventh and twelfth segments of the spinal cord. Thus pain is experienced over these segments bilaterally giving rise to the classical central abdominal pain. As infection increases inflammation of overlying parietal peritoneum occurs and pain is felt locally in the right iliac fossa. Rupture of a gangrenous appendix in a fulminating case may lead to more generalised peritoneal soiling with extension of abdominal tenderness and rigidity of muscles of the entire anterior abdominal wall. Thus tenderness and guarding on examination are at first generalised and not marked. Next they become localised to the right iliac fossa, and finally generalised and very marked if widespread peritonitis develops. In association with inflammation more general features of infection, including malaise, low grade fever, anorexia and flatulence with changes in bowel habit in favour of constipation, are also observed.

Treatment of acute appendicitis is operative, but if a local abscess forms removal of the appendix is usually delayed for six months or so after the infection has subsided. Surgery must be performed when the appendix has perforated and where there is general peritonitis.

Pancreatitis

This is a disorder in which chemical agents, namely pancreatic enzymes, are released and cause irritation of local nerve endings. It occurs chiefly in middle-aged men, especially those who are heavy drinkers. An attack of pain may be precipitated by a heavy meal or alcohol. The pain of acute pancreatitis is agonising and sudden in onset. It is located in the upper abdomen and over the mid-dorsal region, especially to the left side. In both situations its distribution is in the sixth to twelfth thoracic dermatomes, thus the area involved is comparatively large. In association with the pain there is local tenderness and rigidity of muscles of the abdominal wall. Patients also present features of haemodynamic shock with low blood pressure, sweating and pallor, and it is not uncommon for doctors to have difficulty at first in differentiating between this disorder and perforation of a peptic ulcer. Examination may also reveal bradycardia and evidence of hyperglycaemia which produces glycosuria. Estimation of the serum amylase will settle the issue and a past history of peptic ulceration or a previous attack of acute pancreatitis is clearly helpful in reaching a diagnosis. Pancreatitis may also be a progressive disorder of low grade activity and as such give rise to persistent but dull pain over the areas mentioned — particularly in the back. Patients tend to experience mild nausea, occasional episodes of vomiting and may become slightly jaundiced. At times the pain worsens, especially if the patient injudiciously takes excessive food or alcohol. The course of the disorder may be punctuated by attacks of acute pancreatitis.

Acute pancreatitis is self-limiting, usually lasting a few days, and treatment is by means of bed rest with pethidine for pain. In a severe attack the presence of haemodynamic shock with poor peripheral circulation prevents adequate absorption of pethidine by the intramuscular route and, therefore, it is given intravenously as a slow infusion.

Carcinoma of the pancreas

This disease is characterised by paroxysms of very severe epigastric and back pain which is worse when the patient lies on his back. It is associated with anorexia, nausea, rapid weight loss leading to emaciation and to obstructive jaundice which develops in the later stages of the illness. The pain of this condition is so severe that it may lead the patient to commit suicide. Control may be gained by destroying the coeliac plexus using a percutaneous alcohol block, or at open operation when the plexus is destroyed by injecting alcohol into it under direct vision.

Intestinal obstruction

Obstruction of the bowel is most often due to tumour and occurs more frequently in the large than the small bowel. Other intraluminal causes are rare in Britain, though amongst Asian populations obstruction by parasites is well known. Crohn's disease (regional ileitis), a disorder in which there is thickening of the bowel wall, causes extreme narrowing of the lumen of the ileum and can cause obstruction. Similarly though rare nowadays, chronic inflammatory disorders such as tuberculosis can produce the same effect. Bands of tissue (adhesions) which form after surgery, especially where there has been infection, are a common external cause of bowel obstruction. Other causes include herniation through defects in the abdominal wall in the inguinal, femoral or umbilical regions in that order of frequency.

Obstruction of small bowel, the ascending and transverse colon, give rise to central abdominal colic which may be intermittent especially in cases of incomplete obstruction where there may be days or weeks between attacks of pain. Pain from the lower colon is located to the left iliac fossa. This should be remembered because herniation of small bowel in the inguinal region will give rise to central abdominal pain at first and only later, if inflammatory changes develop, to more local symptoms. Obstruction of small bowel is accompanied by vomiting whereas this is much less frequent in large bowel obstruction where, instead, patients become more susceptible to changes in bowel habit and may cease to pass faeces. In the latter situation, which is generally due to tumour growth, obstruction is preceded by alterations in bowel habits perhaps with some blood loss per rectum and more generalised signs such as malaise, weight loss and pallor.

The treatment of intestinal obstruction is surgical and depends upon the site and nature of the disorder, a subject which is beyond the scope of this book.

Diverticulitis

Diverticuli of the descending colon are present in 5 per cent of the population aged 40 years or more and their presence may give rise to colic in the left side of the abdomen. When inflammation occurs abdominal pain is felt chiefly in the left iliac fossa, although on occasions it may occur centrally. In some the pain is colicky, and in others more continuous. Typically it persists for several days and then disappears. In association with pain the patient will have fever and malaise, they may be constipated or have diarrhoea, and slight rectal bleeding is common. Occasionally, especially in the elderly, massive rectal bleeding occurs. Treatment is primarily conservative and only about 10 per cent of patients require surgery. A diet high in fibre, the use of mild aperients and bowel antispasmodics, for example propantheline bromide 15 mg four times daily, is a typical treatment. If pain and rectal bleeding are persistent, if the patient loses weight and becomes anaemic and if a mass is detectable in the left iliac fossa the possibility of a bowel tumour must be considered.

OTHER CAUSES OF ABDOMINAL PAIN

There are many other but less common causes of abdominal pain which are summarised in Table 9.

Table 9 Uncommon causes of abdominal pain

Metabolic causes	Diabetes mellitus
	Porphyria
	Hypokalaemia
	Hyponatraemia
	'Lead poisoning'
	Porphyria
Haematological causes	Henoch-Schöenlein purpura
	Sickle cell anaemia
Neurological causes	Spinal tumours
	Spinal infections
	Multiple sclerosis
	Syphilis (Tabes dorsalis)
Mechanical causes	Intussusception
	Intestinal volvulus
Vascular causes	Rupture of an aortic aneurysm
Infectious causes	Tuberculosis
	Actinomycosis
	Brucellosis
Drugs	Antihypertensive drugs (Ganglion blocking agents)

Psychological aspects of abdominal pain

It is often reasonably easy to differentiate between abdominal pain of organic origin and pain primarily associated with psychological factors. The commonest organic conditions which are simulated by psychologically induced pain, thus causing diagnostic difficulties, are dyspepsia and pain suggesting appendicitis or disease of the large bowel.

Approximately 40 per cent of patients with dyspepsia are free from demonstrable organic lesions. In contrast to patients with a proven peptic ulcer, individuals in this group describe their chief symptoms as a vague rather than a localised upper abdominal discomfort and they have an associated feeling of distension with belching which can be observed during the diagnostic interview. The latter is probably due to frequent swallowing of air (aerophagy) which may also be seen at the same time. Investigations of family circumstances reveal that about half of those afflicted have a parent who had longstanding or frequent episodes of abdominal pain, sometimes organic and sometimes firmly related to psychological factors and this proportion is far in excess of that found amongst a healthy population. Interestingly, a parent's death from a painful abdominal condition occurs prior to the onset of the patient's pain in a quarter of those affected and it may be possible to trace the pain to that time. If so, it is taken as part of the process of mourning in which the patient's physical symptoms act as a protection against excessive mental suffering that might otherwise be present.

In large surveys, where histology of the appendix is studied, about half of all the appendices removed are normal. They are taken from females more often than males in a ratio of about 2 to 1 with the peak age for the former being between 11 and 20 years and the latter between 20 and 30 years. Comparison of histological findings after emergency and 'elective' or delayed appendicectomy where a diagnosis of chronic or 'grumbling' appendicitis has been made, shows that about half the appendices removed as an emergency are normal and over three quarters taken during an elective procedure show no evidence of past or present inflammation. It is only fair to say, however, that some believe that, in the young, appendicular colic without inflammation can lead to signs which are often mistaken for appendicitis leading to unnecessary surgery. Studies of patients with a normal appendix show that significantly more of them are likely to be in need of help for emotional problems and that they are more likely to suffer from recurrent pain after operation than those who have a diseased organ.

A note of caution should be sounded for the studies referred to are based on large groups of patients and it is not always easy to distinguish the symptoms of true appendicitis from psychogenic pain which stimulates it. Thus it is preferable that some normal appendices are removed rather than risk leaving diseased ones.

Irritable colon

In the description of ulcerative colitis it was mentioned that emotional changes have a noticeable effect upon blood flow and motility of the colon. Raised tension, as in states of anger, resentment and hostility, produce hyperaemia, an increase in rhythmic contractions of circular muscle and shortening of longitudinal muscle. These changes occur in the ascending and transverse colon. By contrast, in the descending and sigmoid colon pallor and shortening of muscle occur. In states of dejection, depression and apathy the activity of the colon is reduced, it becomes pallid as mucosal blood flow falls and mucous secretion is reduced too. The physiological changes described are closely related to patients' comments about changes in bowel habit, for example hyperactivity is associated with diarrhoea, and also with pain of colonic origin as part of a common condition known to gastroenterologists as the 'irritable colon syndrome'. This is a chronic disorder usually beginning in the early twenties with a tendency to recur at times of stress. It is more common in women than men and those who suffer from it show evidence of neuroticism, for example, compulsive or phobic symptoms. Most patients have abdominal pain which is sometimes associated with constipation, and at others with diarrhoea. Occasionally only diarrhoea occurs. A number of those who suffer from this disorder undergo unnecessary surgery for suspected appendicitis or a gynaecological disorder, the symptoms of which may be seen to originate from the colon at a later time.

As in the case of other disorders suspected of having a psychological rather than organic basis care must be taken to examine for both possibilities before reaching a diagnosis as the implications for treatment and prognosis are profoundly different for each.

Where a diagnosis of a psychologically determined disorder of bowel function is made treatment should be based on the symptomatic relief of pain and emotional tension using bowel antispasmodics (for example, mebeverine hydrochloride — Colofac), dietary changes to include more roughage, a laxative, (for example, Fybogel), a psychotropic drug, (for example, fluphenazine hydrochloride [0.5 mg] with nortriptyline [10.0 mg] — Motival) and regular daily periods of relaxation. The use of psychological therapy may also be indicated (see Ch. 18).

PAIN IN THE PERINEUM AND RECTUM

The skin of the peri-anal and anal canal below the pectinate line are pain sensitive. Lesions of the rectal mucosa give rise only to vague discomfort.

Pruritis ani

Patients with this condition complain of severe and intractable itching of the anal region. It is associated with a lack of cleanliness and a variety of local conditions, for example, infestation with threadworms, or the presence of haemorrhoids. It is also associated with anxiety. Treatment is by means of control of the causative factor and the use of a local anaesthetic ointment, (3 per cent amethocaine), if the condition is severe.

Proctalgia fugax

This disorder was first described by Maclennan of Glasgow in 1917 in two cases of 'rectal crisis'. The pain is very sudden in onset, short-lasting, severe and stabbing in nature. Usually it halts all activity for a minute or two. The cause of the pain is unknown and examination of anus and rectum will not reveal any abnormality. Those who suffer from proctalgia fugax may be under stress and are said to be of a tense and excitable nature, although the evidence for this is sparse. As the pain is almost always brief treatment is not needed. Reassurance about the benign nature of the condition should be given and if stress is detected its treatment may reduce or abolish the pain. It should also be remembered that patients under stress occasionally present with other pains of variable intensity, duration and sites in the peri-anal and perineal regions without evidence of an organic lesion.

Anal fissure and other local conditions

The patient with an anal fissure gives a history of sharp pain on defaecation, which may be intense and which persists for some time after each bowel action. They may have noticed smearing of the faeces with fresh blood or observed it on toilet paper. Examination reveals marked painful spasm of the anal sphincter muscles (tenesmus), a fissure in the peri-anal skin, and perhaps an associated small skin tag. Fissures are important not only because of the pain they cause but because they may be associated with two major forms of bowel disease — Ulcerative Colitis, and Crohn's disease. Other causes of local pain in the peri-anal region include anal haematomata, which often develop in association with violent physical exertion and are therefore quite common in sportsmen and women, prolapsed thrombosed haemorrhoids, and abscesses.

A simple anal fissure may be treated by the use of mild aperients to avoid constipation, cleanliness, and the application of a local anaesthetic (for example, 3 per cent amethocaine). Intractable cases are treated by stretching the anal sphincter having first given the patient a general anaesthetic. The swiftest treatment of a peri-anal haematoma is release of the blood clot by incision of the skin overlying it.

Carcinoma of the rectum

A squamous cell carcinoma of the anus, or an adenocarcinoma of the rectum invading the anal canal and anus gives rise to severe pain which tends to occur late in the history of the condition. In addition, patients may complain of rectal fullness and will experience tenesmus. The pain associated with carcinoma occurs at the time of defaecation and persists for some time afterwards. The tumour may have the appearance of an anal fissure and there may be slight bleeding also. However, examination reveals more induration than in the case of a simple fissure and inguinal glands may be enlarged. Diagnosis may only be settled finally after a biopsy has been performed and an histological examination carried out. Treatment is surgical.

Prostatitis

Infection of the prostate gland and seminal vesicles gives rise to aching pain felt deep in the pelvis or rectum and a feeling of heaviness in the perineum, low back and legs. The pain may also radiate to the penis. Pain will be exacerbated by sitting, defaecation and rectal examination. If the condition is acute pain will be accompanied by malaise and fever. Frequency occurs when the infection spreads to the bladder. Rectal examination reveals a tender prostate gland and one lobe may be larger than the other, perhaps with an accompanying infection in, and therefore tenderness of, the seminal vesicles.

PAIN IN FEMALE PELVIC ORGANS

Diseases of the organs of the female reproductive tract give rise to pain over a wide area including the lower abdomen, back, perineum, and lower limbs. It is usually experienced above the pubis and lateral to this but does not rise above the level of the iliac crests. Posteriorly pain occurs in the low sacral and gluteal regions. Pain arising from the uterus, cervix, parametria, fallopian tubes and ovaries may be experienced in the lower abdomen alone or in combination with sacral pain. If abdominal pain rises above the level of the iliac crests it is unlikely to be due to a primary disease of the genital organs except in cases where there is free blood in the abdomen (for example, following rupture of an ectopic pregnancy) or peritonitis (for example, following rupture of an abscess in a fallopian tube). Pain may extend into the upper anterior regions of the thighs as in dysmenorrhoea but seldom to other parts of the leg. The most common exception is the occurrence of sciatica caused by invasion of the sacral plexus or sciatic nerve by a malignant tumour (for example, of the cervix). Diseases of the genital organs do not give rise to pain in the high lumbar or other spinal regions. Pain caused by disease of the genital tract will almost always be worse just before menstruation, it increases as the day progresses and often it is diffuse and aching in nature. The patient's history may reveal that its onset dates from the time of pregnancy, labour, or the puerperium.

Acute pain

Acute pain due to diseases of the genital organs or disturbances in their function may be episodic, as in dysmenorrhoea and mid-cycle pain, or constant, as in the case of infections or the development of an ectopic pregnancy. Confusion with acute infection of the appendix is common and therefore it is not surprising that 20 per cent of women submitted to appendicectomy are discovered to have an incorrectly diagnosed gynaecological disorder.

Dysmenorrhoea

Dysmenorrhoea is a common complaint and takes the form of low abdominal central cramp of variable severity occurring during the first 12 to 24 hours of menstruation. It is probably caused by powerful and incoordinated contractions of the uterus and secondary muscle ischaemia. Most of those affected are girls and young women and in many cases dysmenorrhoea disappears after the age of 25 to 30 years — often after childbirth. Usually treatment with simple analgesics is very effective and occasionally bed rest is required. In more intractable cases hormones which inhibit ovulation should be used over a period of several months to give relief. Mid-cycle pain or 'Mittelschmerz' is also physiological in origin and occurs at the time of ovulation in approximately 50 per cent of women. The pain is a cramp or a continuous ache and located in either of the iliac fossae or the hypogastrium. It lasts from 12 to 24 hours and treatment with simple analgesics may be needed.

Infection of the fallopian tubes

A low grade infection of the fallopian tubes and ovaries (salpingo-oöphoritis) gives rise to persistent low backache which is worse prior to menstruation. The patient complains of deep dyspareunia, has a persistent mucopurulent vaginal discharge and heavy, frequent periods. She may first appear at her doctor's surgery complaining of inability to conceive and on examination some tenderness and swelling in the region of the fallopian tubes will be detected. An acute infection or salpingitis produces severe lower abdominal pain, fever and malaise, a blood-stained purulent vaginal discharge, and frequency of micturition. Vaginal examination gives rise to pain and acutely painful swellings may be palpable in the Pouch of Douglas. This condition should not be confused with acute appendicitis, or acute pyelitis, both of which are associated with fever. It may be mistaken for the symptoms of a ruptured ectopic pregnancy or of intestinal obstruction which give rise to severe, acute abdominal pain, but without fever.

The treatment of infections of the female genital tract is a matter for gynaecologists and therefore is not an appropriate topic for inclusion in this book.

Ectopic pregnancy

One in 300 pregnancies occurs outside the uterus, the most common site being one of the fallopian tubes. The commonest cause is damage to a tube which narrows but does not totally obstruct it (for example, following tuberculous salpingitis). At first the patient complains of cramp-like or colicky pain which is unilateral. She will have signs of early pregnancy, namely amenorrhoea and slight breast activity. Examination reveals tenderness over the tubal area, the cervix will be soft, and the uterus slightly enlarged. The tube containing the pregnancy will be palpable, swollen and tender on vaginal examination. If the tube ruptures severe abdominal pain and hypovolaemic shock follows. The abdominal pain becomes generalised and the picture of peritonitis is established. The treatment of the condition is surgical.

Chronic pain

There are several specific causes of chronic pelvic pain including genital prolapse, retroversion of the uterus, endometriosis. cervical infection and adhesions caused by previous infection or surgery in the pelvis. Dyspareunia is intermittent pain experienced during intercourse and might be regarded as chronic intermittent pain.

Cervical infection

Infection of the cervix gives rise to low sacral aching pain which increases as the time for menstruation draws close. The pain may be felt in either iliac fossa, and present as deep dyspareunia. The patient complains of a vaginal discharge and soreness, postcoital or inter-menstrual bleeding, and perhaps dysuria and frequency of micturition also. Referral to a gynaecologist for treatment is recommended.

Dyspareunia

Pain on intercourse has several possible physical causes. They include inflammatory disease in the pelvis, uterine displacement, endometriosis or stenosis of the vaginal entrance. In these conditions pain tends to be experienced only on deep penetration of the vagina but patients who have vaginal stenosis are an exception. Other causes of dyspareunia are psychological and arise as a result of spasm of the introitus of the vagina on attempted intercourse (Vaginismus). The precipitating factors include ignorance of sexual function, fear of intercourse — perhaps as a result of pain on previous occasions — and difficulties in emotional relationships with the spouse or partner. Unlike dyspareunia due to most physical causes pain is experienced when vaginal penetration is attempted. The treatment of dyspareunia is a matter for a gynaecologist if a definite physical abnormality is found. Vaginismus occurring without evidence of physical disease or dysfunction should be treated by sexual counselling. The objectives of treatment are to ensure that the patient has an adequate knowledge of sexual functions, and to teach her and her partner how to overcome anxiety, fear and the resultant pain. This is usually achieved using the method of 'sensate focussing', the details of which will be found in more specialised texts dealing with the management of sexual problems. In addition to attention to specific sexual difficulties the therapist will explore and, if possible, help with other aspects of emotional problems between the couple.

Chronic pelvic pain of unknown origin

Specific causes for continuous or intermittent pelvic pain have been described but there are large numbers of women who haunt doctors' surgeries and gynaecologists' clinics with complaints of chronic aching pain in the lower abdomen and back for which no obvious physical cause is found. These women have attracted considerable attention over the years and a variety of names have been given to their disorder including chronic parametritis, the cervical syndrome, pelvic congestion and several others. Despite the various hypotheses put forward to explain pain none have proved satisfactory so far. However, it has been observed repeatedly that women who experience this form of pain have similar psychological characteristics. They tend to be introverted, prone to anxiousness and to periodic depression. Hysterical elements in the personality are common. Many sufferers have difficulties in forming satisfactory relationships with their husbands and, not surprisingly, sexual difficulties are a major source of feelings of anxiety, anger, guilt and frustration. A thorough physical examination, including laparoscopy, is necessary although it should not reveal any physical abnormality. Remembering that these patients seek desperately for a physical cause for pain initial reassurance that there is no evidence of disease, though not an effective treatment in itself, is usually necessary before any form of psychological investigation will be permitted. Currently, it is believed that this form of pelvic pain is stress-induced, rather like migraine or the irritable bowel syndrome, and it may help treatment to draw an analogy between the patient's pain problem and these conditions as preparation for a psychological approach. There is justification for this approach because there is a growing body of evidence showing that the number of attacks of pelvic pain can be reduced substantially by relatively simple psychotherapy. Success is greatest when a psychiatrist or psychologist works in the gynaecological clinic.

10

Limb pain

Limb pain may arise as a result of disorder of:

1. Joints, bones and muscles.
2. Peripheral nerves.
3. Blood vessels.

PAIN FROM JOINTS

Osteoarthritis

Osteoarthritis is a degenerative condition which affects central and peripheral diarthrodial joints. It is most common in the distal interphalangeal joints of the fingers (50 per cent of all cases) and occurs also in the carpo-metacarpal joints of the thumbs (30 per cent), metatarso-phalangeal joints of the great toes (30 per cent), proximal interphalangeal and metacarpo-phalangeal joints of the fingers (20 per cent), hips (15 per cent), and shoulders, elbows and wrists (5 per cent). It occurs in the cervical spine and lumbar spine too (both 40 per cent of cases). Occasionally it occurs in the acromioclavicular and sternoclavicular joints and may be very troublesome if present in the temporomandibular joints. Osteoarthritis is present in 80 per cent of the population over 55 years of age although only 20 per cent of those affected experience symptoms. Men and women are affected equally. When it presents in early or middle life osteoarthritis is almost always secondary to damage to a joint by injury or disease.

The chief symptoms are pain during or after movement of a joint increasing as the day passes and stiffness, (known as gelling), with loss of function after periods of immobility. Thus there may be difficulty in walking on rising in the morning, or after prolonged rest in a chair. The pain is aching in nature and arises from both the joint and muscles which surround it because they are reflexly thrown into spasm. As a consequence of nerve irritation by osteophytes in the cervical or lumbar spine patients experience brachalgia or sciatica. In the case of osteoarthritis of the hip, pain may occur in both the hip and knee because the nerves supplying each region have a common root of origin. Pain is least severe when joints are kept moving and when the patient is warm. Deformity of the joint is also a characteristic of the disease. For example, Heberden's nodes which develop classically at the distal interphalangeal joints of the fingers or the first interphalangeal joint of the thumb are at first red and painful swellings but later become hard and bony without redness though painful. Movement of an osteoarthritic joint produces a grating sensation, or crepitus, in addition to pain. In some cases an effusion within a joint, for example the knee, will be detectable and produce swelling. Confirmation of osteoarthritis is gained from radiological investigation of affected joints which will reveal narrowing of the joint space, sclerosis of bone ends in which there may be cysts and osteophyte formation.

As most people are only mildly affected symptomatic relief is obtained from simple analgesics and non-steroid anti-inflammatory drugs such as aspirin, and ibuprofen (Brufen) respectively.

Rheumatoid arthritis

In this condition, which differs strikingly from osteoarthritis, there is symmetrical chronic inflammation of small joints: primarily the metacarpo-phalyngeal and proximal interphalangeal joints of the hands and comparable joints in the feet. There are several possible systemic manifestations which include anaemia, neuropathies, vasculitis, subcutaneous nodules, pulmonary and ocular diseases. About three-quarters of those afflicted are young or middle-aged (between the ages of 25 and 55) with women predominating in a ratio of 3 to 1. The onset of rheumatoid arthritis may be preceded by an organic illness or follow a period of emotional stress and for this reason it is often regarded as a psychosomatic disorder. The main symptoms are pain, stiffness and loss of function in the afflicted joints, which include small joints of the hands and feet, the wrists, knees, cervical spine and, at times, the temperomandibular joint. Aching pain predominates and it is associated with stiffness which is worse after periods of immobility, such as sleep or prolonged rest. It is relieved by exercise and warmth. In addition to being painful the joints are swollen and, in contrast to the hard, bony swellings of osteoarthritis, soft or 'boggy'. Deformity of the hands and feet is common and may become extreme requiring surgical correction.

Apart from joint symptoms and other symptomatic effects mentioned, rheumatoid arthritis is associated with significant mental disturbances in many patients for, as might be expected, they are often depressed by the combined effects of chronic pain and disability and by feelings of weakness and malaise that accompany the associated constitutional disturbances. Compared with normal people about half all rheumatoid patients will be depressed and of these 10 to 20 per cent will have severe symptoms. Amongst those who become depressed there is a significantly higher number with premorbid emotional instability than amongst those who do not. Bearing in mind that this chronic painful disease tends to affect young adults more than any other age group, severe emotional problems apart from depression develop because of its physical and social consequences. For example, persistent tiredness reveals to the patient that his or her strength and vigour are substantially reduced. Physical limitations restrict social activities and the patient's life pattern undergoes radical alterations which have the effect of promoting feelings of inferiority and insecurity. They also impair personality development leading to inconsistent behaviour with difficulties in taking criticism, adapting to change and with tendencies to sudden emotional outbursts.

Rheumatoid arthritis is a condition in which treatment by physical and psychological methods is often required. The doctor must help patients retain their independence and social mobility at home and at work as long as possible. Physical treatment has as its basis rest for inflamed joints and the use of anti-inflammatory drugs. Unfortunately these drugs do have side-effects which are unacceptable to patients, for example dyspepsia, and there are dangers associated with their administration to patients with a history of peptic ulceration, cardiac, renal or hepatic disease. Therefore, bearing these points in mind and the fact that there is considerable variation in patient's susceptibility to side-effects, it should be determined, by trial and error, which drug gives the best relief from pain and stiffness with the lowest level of side-effects. In general the newer non-corticosteroidal anti-inflammatory drugs (for example, naproxen—Naprosyn, or azapropazone—Rheumox) are more effective and better tolerated than aspirin or older preparations such as indomethacin (Indocid). If aspirin is considered necessary it may be prescribed as benorylate (Benoral, an aspirin/paracetamol ester), given twice daily (see Chapter 14.) Where simple drugs fail, and this occurs in a relatively small number of patients who are severely affected, phenylbutazone may be prescribed. For very severe cases either corticosteroids or ACTH (adrenocorticotrophic hormone) are used. Surgery involving synovectomy or joint replacement is indicated where the patient's disease is well controlled apart from one or two joints which remain persistently painful and show steady deterioration. Psychological treatment is based upon efforts to help individuals adjust to the physical and social consequences of their disease which may mean developing entirely new ways of life with different goals in terms of work and social achievements. The use of antidepressant therapy is indicated if depressive symptoms are severe and persistent.

Acute gout

This form of arthritis is secondary to a metabolic disorder in which an abnormality of purine biosynthesis, involving the transformation of purines into uric acid, leads to abnormally high levels of uric acid in the blood and to the periarticular deposition of crystals of monosodium urate as a consequence. The latter causes arthritis and renal impairment. Attacks of gout occur most often in middle-aged and elderly men and appear with great rapidity. A variety of factors have been associated with their precipitation and these include over indulgence in foods high in purines, alcohol, starvation diets, trauma, infection and the use of diuretics. The chief symptom is exquisite pain, usually in the first metatarsophalyngeal joint which becomes swollen, purple to red in colour, and hot. The patient may have a raised temperature and anorexia, and examination of blood shows an elevated erythrocyte sedimentation rate and a high serum uric acid level.

If left untreated an attack will last 7 to 14 days but is shortened if the patient is promptly given non-corticosteroid anti-inflammatory drugs (see Chapter 14).

The painful shoulder

There are several disorders which give rise to pain in the region of the shoulder and which are caused by damage to muscle tendons or their sheaths. Aching pain which worsens on external rotation of the arm without evidence of radiological changes in the bone sometimes follows unaccustomed exercise. This may be due to synovitis of the long head of biceps tendon sheath as it lies in the bicipital groove on the lateral aspect of the humerus. The pain is well localised and associated with tenderness on pressure over the groove and the condition may last for several weeks or months. More generalised pain of an aching nature occurs in the region of the shoulder joint where calcific deposits are present in the tendons of muscles which arise from the scapula and pass to their insertion in the region of the joint. In addition to pain there is limitation of movement, especially if the patient attempts to abduct the arm at the shoulder and, in particular, as it moves between 70° and 130° of abduction. The latter sign is also typical of a specific supraspinatus tendinitis. In the elderly either syndrome may lead to more generalised pain or stiffness in the arm which is slow to clear and this condition, which is called a 'frozen shoulder', may occur spontaneously or when the arm is allowed to remain immobilised for a time as may happen, though it should not, following a stroke which produces hemiplegia.

Treatment of all these disorders involves local heat, gentle exercise, and perhaps local injections of cortico-steroids in resistent cases.

BONE PAIN

Sensitivity to noxious stimuli resides in the periosteum of bone as is evident from consideration of the fact that burr holes can be cut in the skull with a hand operated or motorised drill in conscious patients. They do not experience pain unless there is traction or pressure upon the periosteum which is, therefore, anaesthetised. Bone pain originates from the effects of trauma, inflammation, or tumour infiltration of periosteum. In addition it also occurs in disorders of bone metabolism, including osteomalacia and senile osteoporosis. Distortion of bone in Paget's disease, as with other conditions that have this effect, produces abnormal stresses and strains upon ligaments and joints which cause pain to arise from them. Paget's disease may also lead to direct compression of nerves as the bone thickens and this too produces pain.

MUSCLE PAIN

The commonest cause of muscle pain is 'tearing' of muscles which in reality means damage to their tendinous fibres of origin from, or their insertions into, bone. It is also caused quite often by physiologically or pathologically induced ischaemia. 'Tennis elbow' is a common example of pain due to damage at the origin of muscle fibres from bone. In this condition pain is located accurately to the lateral epicondyle of humerus where fibres of forearm muscles are attached. Trauma is the usual cause and pain is provoked by supination of the forearm and hand as in wringing wet clothing. The condition is self-limiting and responds to rest though it often persists for several months. Local injections of corticosteroids into the site of origin of the muscles are used to bring relief in resistant cases.

Pain due to ischaemia and venostasis

Ischaemic pain arising from muscles is due to hypoxia in degenerative vascular disorders which include atherosclerosis, thromboangitis obliterans, arterial thrombosis and embolism. It may also occur in severe anaemia and myxoedema. The pain is due to accumulation of the products of anaerobic respiration and it disappears either when the work of the muscle decreases or when adequate oxygenation of tissues is achieved permitting metabolism to return to normal. This occurs when any obstruction to blood flow is relieved as in embolectomy or arterial disobliteration, where vascular dilation is achieved by the use of drugs such as phenoxybenzamine, or following sympathectomy, though the latter dilates blood vessels in the skin rather more than in the muscles. Ischaemic pains are often described as cramps or knotting of muscles. Where degenerative arterial disease is present in the branches of the abdominal aorta supplying the lower limbs, blood flow is reduced to such a low level that exercise leads to greater demands for oxygen than can be supplied. Therefore, the speed with which pain develops depends upon the efficiency of the arterial circulation. Patients are able to walk only a limited distance after which they develop pain. This disappears with rest only to reappear on further activity and is known as intermittent claudication. Claudication is commonest in the lower limbs where it occurs chiefly in the muscles of the calf and occasionally in the buttocks. Clinicians use the 'claudication distance' and its changes with time as a rough guide to the progression of the disease. When blood flow is severely hampered by arterial disease pain occurs at rest, particularly if the affected limbs is warm and its metabolism exceeds the rate at which oxygen arrives at the tissues in amounts required by their metabolic processes. This is not the only reason, however, for severe deep pain may also be produced as a result of ischaemia in peripheral nerves due to low blood flow in the vasa nervorum. Ischaemic neuritis produces a severe burning pain which is unrelieved by rest and which is associated with hyperaesthesia or analgesia in appropriate dermatomes.

Ischaemic neuritis is probably irreversible and treatment of pain is by means of analgesic drugs although these vary in their effectiveness from person to person. However, rest pain may be relieved by the removal or by-passing of a block within a major artery, or by the control of infection. In less severe cases reduction of plasma viscosity may help as may the improvement of the microcirculation using low molecular weight dextran. There is interest also in the use of Praxilene (naftidrofuryl) which is said to stimulate tissue respiration and prevent or reduce the accumulation of pain producing tissue metabolities.

Occlusion of a major artery gives rise to sudden and very severe pain in the limb. The affected area becomes white, cold and pulseless, and paraesthesia may be experienced. This condition requires surgical treatment within 24 hours. In the meantime the limb should be kept at rest and cool to reduce the metabolic needs of the tissues.

In addition to inadequacies of arterial blood flow in relatively large vessels pain may also result from disorders of circulation through smaller arterioles. This situation occurs in Raynaud's Disease. The condition is most common amongst young women who are usually susceptible to the effects of low temperature which leads to constriction of arterioles in the fingers and toes. The mechanism for this is uncertain, though it is thought to be due to alteration in activity of the sympathetic part of the autonomic nervous system. As a result of reduced blood flow in the fingers and toes they become white, numb and painful. During recovery skin colour changes from blue to red as the area becomes hyperaemic and at the same time the skin becomes very warm. Pain is accentuated at the onset of the process. Apart from this unusual physiological response to low temperatures the phenomenon described may also occur in a number of diseases which include rheumatoid arthritis, polyarteritis nodosa and scleroderma. In the case of a patient with rheumatoid arthritis the presence of severe and persistent Raynaud's phenomena is taken as a possible indication of scleroderma. The symptoms of Raynaud's Disease may be reduced or abolished by the use of a drug which dilates peripheral blood vessels (for example, bamethan sulphate—Vasculit), but such agents should be used with caution as they are contra-indicated in patients with a history of myocardial infarction or angina.

Lower limb pains, heavy and aching in nature, are common in individuals with varicose veins. In women the pain is worse premenstrually and in all cases it is reduced or completely relieved either by rest with the feet elevated above the level of the pelvis and by the wearing of elastic stockings. These measures effectively reduce or prevent venostasis and distension of veins which, together with tissue oedema, give rise to pain. More acute and well localised pains occur with thrombophlebitis or the appearance of a varicose ulcer.

THE CERVICOBRACHIAL SYNDROME

As the neurovascular bundle enters the arm through an area bounded by the 1st rib posteriorly, and the clavicle anteriorly, its vascular and nervous elements may be distorted, or compressed, by the scalene muscles, the tendon of insertion of pectoralis minor, an extension of the transverse process of the 7th cervical vertebra (cervical rib), or an abnormality of the 1st rib. These anomalies may ultimately lead to pain in the arm but often this is delayed until the middle years of life and is most common in women. Complaints are made of dull pain in the forearm and ulna border of the hand and the symptom is worsened by carrying heavy loads, for example a loaded shopping basket. Numbness, tingling and muscle wasting occur in the distribution of the nerve supplied by the 8th cervical and first thoracic nerve roots, (chiefly the ulnar nerve), and the pulse on the affected side may be reduced in amplitude either permanently or on deliberate traction of the arm. Occasionally Raynaud's phenomenon is present.

Treatment of the condition involves surgery directed towards correction of the anatomical anomaly.

PAIN ARISING FROM PERIPHERAL NERVES

Injury to peripheral nerves or their entrapment as they pass through or beneath fascial thickenings or ligaments are relatively common causes of pain, though there are many others (see Table 10). Neuropathic pain is either a steady burning experience, a shooting sensation, or at worst an indescribable feeling of discomfort or unpleasantness. It is accompanied by evidence of damage to neuronal conduction which includes numbness, hypoaesthesia, hyper-

Table 10 Examples of causes of pain arising from peripheral nerves

Nerve compression	Arm and hand	Cervical rib syndrome Ulnar neuritis Carpal tunnel syndrome
	Trunk	Nerve entrapment (e.g. meralgia paraesthetica)
	Leg and foot	Nerve entrapment at ankle Plantar digital neuroma
Partial or complete division of a nerve		Causalgia Amputation stump neuroma
Metabolic nerve injury and ischaemia		Diabetic neuropathy Alcoholic polyneuritis Acute infective polyneuritis Limb arteriosclerosis Hypothyroidism
Neural manifestations of infectious diseases		Measles Syphilis Leprosy

aesthesia and muscle weakness or total paralysis. Trophic changes in muscles, bone and skin are also seen from time to time.

Causalgia

The term causalgia was coined by Dr Weir Mitchell in 1864 to describe the intense burning pain that may follow partial nerve damage which generally occurs as the result of an accident or, occasionally, after a surgical operation upon a peripheral nerve. The pain appears in only 2–5 per cent of injuries and is present in most cases almost immediately after injury, although in some it is delayed for weeks or months. In the affected region there is an alteration in sweating and temperature regulation and as a consequence the skin becomes dry, warm and shiny due to alterations in the activity of the autonomic nervous system. These appear to involve stimulation of sprouting axons in the damaged nerve fibres by noradrenaline released from active sympathetic nerve fibres in the same area. The extent of the physiological changes is usually greater than the area supplied by the damaged somatic nerve, or nerves. There is muscle wasting, loss of power and pain which is intensified enormously by touching the affected part lightly. In order to protect themselves against the latter patients wear a glove or wrap the limb firmly, perhaps splinting it in some way, to prevent movement which in itself may cause pain. Raised emotional tension increases pain and this is thought to be due to alterations in activity of the autonomic nervous system at centres which are also concerned with the control of emotional activity. The treatment of choice is a permanent sympathetic ganglion block or surgical sympathectomy. Recently it has been shown that blocking sympathetic activity by a local infusion of guanethidine distal to a cuff on the affected limb also abolishes pain, usually for long periods. This procedure should only be carried out in hospital by those experienced in parenteral use of such drugs.

Causalgia is one member of a group of disorders known as reflex sympathetic dystrophies, or algodystrophies, and all give rise to hyperpathia and allodynia. All tissues in the affected area, including bones, waste, and there is evidence of abnormal sympathetic control, including vasomotor changes and inappropriate sweating. The effects of the disorders appear to extend into the spinal cord and from there to the periphery via sympathetic nerves. They respond to a block of sympathetic activity. The causes of these conditions include nerve damage, fractures of the small bones of the hand or foot (for example, a scaphoid fracture), sprains, or superficial thrombophlebitis. Rarely, the cause is a lesion in the central nervous system.

Nerve entrapment in the upper arm

In the upper arm two conditions predominate—ulnar neuritis and the carpal tunnel syndrome.

Ulnar neuritis

This disorder is characterised by pain, numbness and tingling in the sensory distribution of the ulnar nerve in the hand which covers the palm on the ulnar side of the hand, the little finger and the ulnar half of the ring finger. The interosseous and hypothenar muscles which are also supplied by the ulnar nerve may be wasted and weak. Symptoms tend to be worse on awakening from sleep and it is thought that this is due to the effect of sleeping with the elbow flexed which increases compression of the nerve. The condition may be caused by thickening of the band of fascia which keeps the ulnar nerve in place as it passes behind the medial epicondyle of the humerus. Treatment is to cut this at operation and, in some cases, the nerve is transposed to lie anteriorly to ensure that there is no possibility of recurrence. The condition may also be due to compression of the nerve as it passes between the heads of the flexor carpi ulnaris muscle which are separated to free the nerve.

The carpal tunnel syndrome

In this disorder the median nerve is compressed as it lies beneath the flexor retinaculum in the carpal tunnel at the wrist. Numbness, tingling and pain occur in the sensory distribution of the median nerve which supplies the remainder of the area of the palm and palmer surface of the fingers not supplied by the ulnar nerve (see above), together with the dorsal surfaces of the tips of the index, middle fingers and radial half of the tip of the ring finger. The thenar muscles, and especially adductor policis brevis, are weak and wasted and in chronic cases the grip is correspondingly poor. Tingling is provoked by tapping or pressing over the carpal tunnel, (Tinels's sign), and pain is worse at night or after exercise. The condition affects young and middle-aged women far more often than men. The reason for the appearance of the disorder is not always clear, though it may be that the tunnel is more often small in relation to the bulk of its contents in women. Water retention, as in the pre-menstrual period and in conditions such as myxoedema, lead to the appearance or exacerbation of symptoms. The carpal tunnel syndrome may also appear in association with arthritis of the wrist joint or after fractures, in other words in conditions which reduce the size of the carpal tunnel. At times it appears during pregnancy and in haemophilia. Sixty per cent of patients respond to conservative treatment which involves resting the affected part. A night splint for the wrist used over a period of a month is recommended for patients who do not respond to this simple measure. Surgical treatment involves decompression of the contents of the canal by division of the tissues forming its roof. At operation thickening of the synoveum of the tendon sheaths in the canal is a constant feature.

Meralgia paresthetica

This is a condition which presents with a burning pain, numbness and tingling over the antero-lateral aspects of the thigh due to compression of lateral femoral cutaneous nerve at one of several points on its course after it emerges from behind the lateral border of the psoas muscle on the posterior abdominal wall, and its ultimate entry into the tissues of the thigh by passage through the inguinal ligament. Within the abdomen it may be compressed by tumour masses, or in the pelvis by the uterus where the nerve crosses the iliacus muscle. It may also be damaged as it crosses the anterior part of the iliac crest and perforates the inguinal ligament. Occasionally damage to the nerve occurs when an intramuscular injection is given into the lateral aspect of the thigh. Treatment of the condition is by means of repeated local anaesthetic block just below the point where the nerve enters the thigh and occasionally it is avulsed deliberately at operation, though this does not completely guarantee relief.

Nerve entrapment at the ankle

The posterior tibial nerve may be compressed beneath the flexor retinaculum of the foot at its point of division into the medial and lateral plantar nerves. The symptoms of the condition closely resemble those of the carpal tunnel syndrome and its treatment is similar.

PAINFUL HEEL

Pain in the region of the heel radiating beneath the foot may be the result of plantar fasciitis, which is a condition that can arise spontaneously or in association with ankylosing spondylitis, rheumatoid arthritis, gonococcal infection and Reiter's disease. Pain may also be due to an unrecognised fracture of the calcaneum, especially in those who have newly entered the Armed Forces where marching and drill are a prominent aspect of training.

PAINFUL FOOT

Marching, or a long walk in someone unaccustomed to such exercise, may produce a stress fracture of a metatarsal bone, (a March fracture). Tenderness is local and the fracture is seen on X-ray examination. On rare occasions pain may be due to a neuroma on a plantar digital nerve. It is most likely to occur on the nerve running between the heads of the 1st and 2nd metatarsal bones and it gives rise to a stabbing pain which radiates either to the toe or to the leg. Tenderness is present locally at the site of the neuroma and treatment is removal by surgical operation.

LIMB PAINS IN TABES DORSALIS

In the tertiary stage of a syphilitic infection a patient may develop demyelination in the dorsal nerve roots and dorsal ascending columns of the spinal cord. The functions served by the latter are vibration and joint position sense and part of the sensation of touch. Thus, in tabes dorsalis postural sense and the sense of vibration are absent. Pain, which is normally felt after squeezing the Achilles tendon or testicles (deep pain) is absent. Ability to experience pain on noxious stimulation of the central area of the face, front of the chest, inner arms, outer aspect of the legs, soles of the feet and in the perianal region disappears. However, spontaneous pain occurs and is sharp or stabbing in nature and often called 'lightning pain'. Each attack is brief lasting a few seconds and pain shifts from place to place on different occasions. It is worse in wet weather and when the patient has an infection. The pains may be experienced in all limbs and in the territory of the trigeminal nerve also. At times patients also experience severe burning pain in the feet, pain in the distribution of the sciatic nerve or 'girdle pains' which encircle the chest or abdomen. Lightning pain may be elicited by noxious stimulation but interestingly there is a delay in experiencing it and presumably this is a reflection of the effect of damage to the posterior columns.

Treatment with carbamazepine (Tegretol) may bring complete relief.

PAIN IN DIABETES MELLITUS

The most common signs of neuropathy in diabetes mellitus are loss of tendon reflexes and vibration sense in the lower limbs, but it may also give rise to very severe burning pain in the legs, especially the calves. At times there is only pain and weakness with tenderness on gentle squeezing of the muscles. The origin of the disorder is thought to lie in reduction of blood flow in the vascular supply of the nerves, the vasa nervorum, secondary to degenerative changes in major blood vessels. When the blood supply is barely sufficient to maintain normal function of the nerves and local infection is present, demands of tissues for oxygen increase beyond the capacity of the vascular system to supply it and the symptoms of neuropathy appear but can be reversed by appropriate treatment of the infection. The diagnosis is confirmed by gaining proof of the presence of diabetes mellitus. The symptoms of diabetic neuritis can be distinguished from those due to vascular occlusion in major vessels by confirming that peripheral pulses are present proximally and distally in the limbs. The outlook for patients with diabetic neuropathy is good if the primary condition responds well to antidiabetic treatment, or where infection if present is treated successfully. The outlook is also good where there is a mild degree of generalised arteriopathy.

LIMB PAIN AND ALCOHOLISM

Degenerative changes affecting the nervous system in chronic alcoholism are seen mostly in middle aged men. They affect the brain, somatic peripheral nerves and autonomic nervous system. Patients with alcoholic neuritis at an early stage of development complain of numbness, tingling and pain in the hands and feet. The pain is often severe and burning in nature, or 'like flesh being torn from the bones'. Cramps occur in the calves, especially at night, and later both motor and sensory changes are found. Wrist and foot drop, and muscle wasting, may develop especially in the periphery of the limbs. All sensation is reduced and, although anaesthesia or hypoaesthesia can be demonstrated in the skin, muscles are painful to the touch and severe pain may be experienced if the examiner scratches the soles of the patient's feet. Tendon reflexes are diminished or lost.

The cause of alcoholic neuritis is uncertain. but it is thought to arise as a result of a diet lacking vitamins, especially those of the B group. Treatment involves complete withdrawal of alcohol, rest, and the adminstration of vitamins of the B group (Multivite). In mild cases complete recovery may take place, but in those where the disorder is advanced it takes months or may be incomplete.

PHANTOM LIMB PAIN

It was stated earlier that much of our incoming sensory information is dealt with by specific areas in the post-central cortex and in a way that permits the construction of a senory map or homunculus. As a result each of us has an internal 'image' which is representative of our physical selves and it is known as 'the body image'. This becomes distorted in certain forms of epilepsy, in schizophrenia at times, and in normal life on waking from sleep, or in specially contrived conditions where individuals are deprived of the usual amounts of sensory information from their environment.

Loss of part of the body, such as a limb or breast, is often associated with persistence of that part of the body image for sometime afterwards although eventually the 'phantom' of the part tends to shrink and disappear. In about 3 per cent of individuals who undergo amputation of a limb persistent disagreeable sensations or pain, which is often very severe and described as tightness or bursting, are associated with the phantom. In up to about 13 per cent of cases such symptoms occur but are only temporary. Phantom pain is sometimes present together with pain in the amputation stump, but this is by no means always the case.

It is of interest that those who suffer from persistent pain in a phantom limb have certain characteristics in common in terms of events preceding amputation, the nature of the amputation, and their emotional constitution. They often give a history of prolonged physical disability or disease of the limb, usually a painful one, before amputation takes place. For example, there may have been chronic osteomyelitis or, for some reason, several surgical operations. Others tell of very sudden loss of the limb in emotionally traumatic circumstances as in warfare or industrial and road traffic accidents. Those who undergo amputation and develop a painful phantom limb often appear to have a rigid and self-reliant personality with a greater number of previous episodes of depressive illness than those who do not develop persistent symptoms. Thus, to some extent the development of pain problems may be anticipated and pre-operative measures designed to reduce severe post-operative pains can be taken.

Not only does the loss of a limb involve relearning of motor skills, but it also leads to the development of grief at loss of part of the body. This is characterised by depression of mood, tension, poor concentration, self-blame, restless hyperactivity, insomnia and jealousy of others who are normal. Pre-operative counselling of the patient and the family by members of the medical profession and by emotionally well adjusted people who have undergone amputation has been found to be useful because it reduces the intensity of the amputee's response to the loss.

Emotion may also affect the intensity of phantom limb pain just as in the case of pain arising from damage to physically intact parts of the body with the result that increased pain occurs in situations of heightened anxiety, where there is open anger and especially where there is suppressed hostility.

In many cases the phantom and pain disappear without treatment after some months have passed. Where they persist electrical cutaneous stimulation over the stump has proved effective in about half of those treated. Pain in an amputation stump is often due to the formation of a neuroma at the end of a divided nerve and where the latter becomes adherent to the skin, or to moving structures within the stump. Conservative measures for relief include percussion of the neuroma with a small hammer, the use of friction or a cold spray, all of which may well diminish pain for a time. Eventually, however, it is likely that clean excision of the neuroma will be required. The production of local anaesthesia by nerve blocking or cordotomy is not favoured as an anaesthetised limb stump may well be damaged if a prosthesis is worn.

11

Pain, emotion and physical symptoms

It is not generally appreciated that pain is a common complaint amongst emotionally disturbed people, although its occurrence in them rivals the frequency with which it appears in physical diseases. It has been found in general hospitals that of all patients attending medical out-patient clinics three quarters are likely to have pain, and about one third of them may be expected to have an emotional disorder too. A little more than half the attenders at a general practitioner's surgery have emotional disturbances and of these between one third and a half will complain of pain. At first it may seem surprising that pain should be such a prominent symptom amongst the mentally ill until it is remembered that pain is a subjective experience heavily laden with emotional elements. Moreover, because pain is so wellknown to everyone, and because its presence is generally linked solely with physical disease and injury, it is easy to understand why it should appear amongst those taking on the mantle of physical ill health although they do not have clear evidence of a physical basis for their complaints.

Pain, emotion and physical disorders are linked in three ways:

1. Painful physical diseases or injuries produce emotional changes (somatopsychic problems).
2. Pain occurs in physical diseases assumed to be initiated and maintained chiefly by psychological factors (psychosomatic disorders).
3. Pain occurs in mental disorders although physical causes for it are absent.

THE EMOTIONAL CONSEQUENCES OF PAIN IN PHYSICAL ILLNESS

Changes in emotion occurring amongst those in pain result from the combined effects of the physical and social consequences of the disorder giving rise to it and the influence of personality. The effects of acute pain of relatively short duration differ from those of chronic pain. The former raises levels of anxiety reflected in the urgent search for a remedy, preoccuption with the cause of the pain and reduced levels of tolerance for noise and other sensory stimuli which are regarded as 'irritating'. Capacity for sustained concentration is impaired, judgement may become faulty, and relationships with others strained.

Chronic illness is contemplated with anxiety as many of those affected are uncertain of their fate, fear prolonged disability and even death, and are often apprehensive about the possibility of further suffering before life ends. Pain, when present, tends to accentuate these anxieties but mostly the sufferer is concerned about whether or not relief is possible. At times attempts to relieve chronic pain are only partially successful or even unsuccessful which increases patients' anxiety considerably. Drugs of increasing potency, or perhaps surgical procedures, are used to gain control bringing with them side-effects which add to the level of misery. Powerful analgesic drugs can cause reduced awareness and lowering of the powers of concentration, and surgical treatments such as nerve blocks and sections relieve pain but may cause unacceptable anaesthesia, dysaesthesia, failure of bladder function, limb paralysis and other unpleasant sequelae. The nature of the disorder has its own effects too. Chronic benign conditions may not be associted with the prospect of death as in the case of malignancy, but both give rise to fear and depression which follows the initial phase of disbelief and which precedes the final acceptance of irreversible changes, a life of disability or the inevitable termination of life itself. Finally, many diseases produce symptoms other than pain which are the cause of great distress and these include vomiting, diarrhoea, dyspnoea and itching.

Chronic pain leads to withdrawal from social contact and a greater level of introspection than is normally present. The fact that many chronic diseases lessen physical mobility accentuates this reducing an individual's contact with his friends and acquaintances outside the family still further. Neurotic behaviour, including excessive preoccupation with genuine symptoms, anxiety or depression, may appear as the person attempts to come to terms with the problems he has to face, and in some an increase in their consumption of alcohol, or frank alcoholism may develop. There is a significant association between suicide and chronic painful illnesses especially in older men. The clinical picture is flavoured be premorbid personality traits and the way a patient copes with his or her difficulties follows a pattern set in earlier life. In some cases this means a tendency to become more dependent on others than is really necessary, and in others the exhibition of bravura, or the development of depression. There is an increase in complaints about physical discomforts and symptoms that would be ignored or played down at times of better health representing a response to the unpleasant emotional feelings aroused by the illness and preoccupation with such symptoms is greatest amongst patients with pain. Although it seems natural to be absorbed by suffering when it is inescapable and almost constant, even threatening life itself, the level of self-interest varies between individuals. It has been proposed that preoccupation with symptoms is a form of defence in which the sufferer's focus of interest is diverted from the worst emotional consequences of the threats posed by the disease.

PAIN AND PSYCHOSOMATIC DISORDERS

It is obvious that every form of illness has emotional aspects but in certain instances that the disease process is initiated or prolonged by disturbances of emotional life. The cerebral cortex is concerned with the registration and interpretation of information entering the higher centres of the central nervous system, and also with subsequent responses to it. The limbic system, the site of generation of emotional responses, has cortical elements which are linked with the autonomic nervous system and endocrine glands. Under normal circumstances there is a functional balance or harmony between them, but disturbances of emotion produce obvious physical effects mediated by the autonomic system. For example, if emotion is suddenly aroused as in fright, there are alterations in heart rate, respiratory rate, sweating and gastro-intestinal function. More subtle and more extended physiological responses to emotional changes are manifest as disorders of the skin, musculoskeletal, respiratory and gastro-intestinal, cardiovascular and other systems of the body, and these may be prolonged or recurrent depending on the nature and duration of the precipitating stresses. Familiar and common examples of conditions in which such physiological changes occur include giant urticaria, asthma, peptic ulceration and migraine. Those who suffer from psychosomatic illness exhibit certain characteristics, including a strong possibility of the same type of illness occurring in relatives, or a personal history of more than one psychosomatic disorder. Psychosomatic disorders tend to be intermittent, appearing at times of stress, which is defined as the result of circumstances which pose a threat to the emotional integrity of the individual. Stresses arise out of those events in life which are emotionally highly significant but not necessarily unpleasant, as in the case of marriage or the birth of a child. Distress brought about by the death of a close relative or friend, changes in employment, financial disaster and retirement are unpleasant events that may be associated with precipitation or recrudescence of the condition. Most patients, though perhaps not all at first, appreciate the relationship between emotional life and a predisposition to the particular physical condition from which he or she suffers. Only a small number of these disorders are associated with pain, as in the case of migraine and variants of it, angina, gastric disorders and disturbances of bowel function, such as colitis. In each case the link between emotion and physiological function soon becomes obvious both to the doctor and the patient.

This brief account of the physical responses to changes in emotion gives the impression they are specific to each individual and the members of the families who suffer them. In other words the development of migraine, for example, is one person's way of responding to emotional stress and strain, whereas another develops symptoms of a peptic ulcer, and a third ulcerative colitis. This way of responding to the pressures of life is generally understood by the sufferer and his doctor as both are able to link cause and effect without difficulty and to establish a relationship through the treatment of physical symptoms which not only sustains the patient but perhaps leads to discussion about, and relief of the stressful factors causing them. This is not so when complaints of pain and other symptoms are made in the absence of physical abnormality, a situation in which all too often the patient is rejected by doctors, many of whom seem able to accept pain in their patients only when there is a physical basis for it. From the patient's point of view there is usually a desperate need to find a physical explanation and there is abrupt rejection of any suggestion that psychological factors play a major role in the genesis of their symptoms. Thus both doctors and patients seem to find the presence of pain without disease or injury a major objection and an obstruction to appropriate treatment, having failed to realise or accept that pain can be produced by psychological mechanisms alone.

PAIN WITHOUT AN OBVIOUS PHYSICAL CAUSE

Pains have different sensory qualities, associated behaviours vary and their origins lie in some form of disease process, injury, physiological dysfunction, disturbance of emotion, or situations in which pain behaviour is reinforced. Often more than one of these potential causes are present and clearly the balance of psychological and psychic elements must vary from case to case. Therefore, it is unwise to separate pain into 'organic' and 'functional' types, especially because the latter is often interpreted as an indication of deliberate falsification of symptoms or their unreasonable exaggeration, with patients being told that their pain is 'imaginary'; a term used very commonly and carelessly. As a result of doctors' dislike of 'deceitful or dishonest patients' such individuals are often rejected rather than examined with a view to determining why they took the major step of going to a doctor to complain about their plan. The term 'psychogenic' has been used to describe pain states in which psychological factors are the chief element in their generation of maintenance, but its use has been heavily criticised recently because of the unfortunate connotations it seems to arouse in those who fail to understand the possible origins of such states. Therefore, to avoid confusion it is suggested that the shorthand terms 'organic' and 'psychogenic or functional', be discarded in favour of a broader description of any pain state. Thus, one might describe pain arising from tissue injury as having one of several emotional and behavioural elements, or a pain state without an obvious physical cause as being heavily loaded with certain behavioural and psychological aspects. Undoubtedly the reader will regard this as a cumbersome way of dealing with the problem but it does have the virtue of greater accuracy and, importantly, it is less likely to lead to rejection of patients and aggravation of their distress by the use of misleading statements of the following type, 'your pain is all in your mind, it's in your imagination'. The reader's problem of differentiating between the parts played by psychological and organic factors in any given painful disorder should be helped by reference to Table 11.

The onset of pain with prominent psychological characterisitics is seldom easy to define and it may have been present intermittently or continuously for several years. Only when linked to acute major mental disorders, for example depression or schizophrenia, is the pain likely to be shortlived. In those who have pain related to abnormalities of personality or a chronic neurosis the history will extend over a period of months or years. More women than men suffer this type of pain which parallels the greater incidence of neurotic disorders amongst them. Most patients come from the lower socio-economic groups in the community perhaps because amongst the less will educated, appreciation of, or acceptance of emotional difficulties is less than that of physical disorders. Pain strongly influenced by psychological factors occurs with greater frequency in some parts of the body than in others. Fifty to sixty per cent of

Table 11 Indications of physical and physiological elements in pain states

Indications of marked physical elements in a pain state	Indications of marked psychological and behavioural elements in a pain state
Onset. Usually clearcut.	Vague or uncertain. Often no Precipitating factor.
Nature. Well recognised characteristics, e.g. colic, pain of myocardial infarction. Interferes with sleep.	Often not well described. May be a discrepancy between severity described and behaviour. Often not present during night hours.
Site. Usually recognised by its relation to injury or disease or to its site if referred.	Ill-defined in some cases. In others may occur at site of previous tissue damage (trauma, surgery etc). More often on left side of body.
Increased by movement, palpation etc.	Increased by wide range of stimuli or, unchanged by any stimulus. May change in relation to mood variation.
Relieved by physical means, i.e. rest, analgesics, surgery etc.	Anxiolytic drugs, alcohol and other methods of reducing emotional tension. Often said to be unresponsive to any treatment.
Other features. Psychological factors prominent as secondary changes, i.e. development of depression or anxiety.	Commonly permorbid history of neurotic traits or mental illness. The latter are usually neurotic disorders.

patients complain of pain in the region of the head and face. Abdominal and chest pain is less common, accounting for about 10–20 per cent of suffering, with the anterior trunk and lower back being the most common sites for it. Pain occurs least in the limbs or genitalia. For reasons that are not understood it is commoner in the left half of the body. The pain may be described clearly but more often it is vague, ill-localised and inconstant in position. Contrary to popular belief only a minority of patients describe their pain in bizarre terms, or complex ways, and the vividness of descriptions tends to be related mainly to personality. The pain seldom wakens patients at night and its severity may be so obviously connected to levels of emotional tension that this has been noticed even by the patient. Analgesic drugs are unreliable in bringing relief, whereas tranquillisers, hypnotics and alcohol may be effective. The pain is often said to be present during interview and examination and yet the patient's behaviour gives no outward sign of the level of suffering described. This discrepancy is marked at times and a potent source of irritation to some doctors! Careful physical examination shows that its distribution does not bear a close relation to the sensory dermatomes of the body, or to accepted areas where referred pain occurs.

Where pain has been a longstanding problem past history may reveal facts. Patients' relatives show a greater than normal tendency to have had persistent painful illnesses and indeed, at times, the patient's own symptoms are similar to those experienced by the relative in question. Their own histories are littered with frequent consultations with the family doctor and punctuated by referrals to medical, surgical, gynaecological or dental specialists who carry out intensive investigations, sometimes leading to needless surgical operations, or to other potentially hazardous treatments. It should be remembered that injudicious remarks about symptoms that might be present and vague suggestions of some serious but as yet undiscovered problem fuel patients' desires for yet more consultations and so perpetuate unnecessary involvement of increasing numbers of doctors.

The main responsibility for diagnosis clearly lies with family doctors and, indeed, it is probable that only a minority of patients reach hospital specialists, but unfortunately too few receive expert psychiatric help, especially during the early stages of their disorder.

12

Pain and mental illness

Chronic pain amongst those who are emotionally disturbed is associated chiefly with the neuroses and disorders of personality development.

Neuroses are disorders of emotion in which psychological and physical symptoms occur and which are similar in nature if not in scale to the experiences of normal people exposed to stress. The difference in quality between a neurotic reaction and normality is difficult to make at times as one shades imperceptibly into the other, but it is accepted that a neurosis is present when the response to stress is excessive in relation to the stimulus which provoked it and when it is unduly prolonged after the stimulus has ceased to operate. Most patients who develop neuroses are aware of the relation between stress and their emotional response to it and their interpretation of the reality of the world around them is not seriously disturbed. The neuroses are not the result of any structural or metabolic defect in the brain and thus differ from those disorders of mental life known as the organic psychoses which arise in this way.

The neuroses most commonly associated with psychogenic pain are:

1. Anxiety
2. Depression
3. Hypochondriasis
4. Hysteria

Often more than one of the elements 1–4 are present together for example, anxiety and depressive symptoms are frequently paired, as are depression and hypochondriasis and a sense of inner tension or strain accompanies all forms of disturbance to some extent.

In the Glossary of Mental Disorders included in the International Classification of Diseases the psychoses include 'those conditions in which impairment of mental functions developed to a degree that interferes grossly with insight, ability to meet some of the ordinary demands of life, or adequate contact with reality'. Included under this heading are:

1. Psychoses arising from a physical disease, injury or degenerative condition of the brain, or secondary to systemic diseases affecting the function of brain (the organic psychoses).

2. Psychoses which do not have any definite origin in disturbances of the brain function, although these may be strongly suspected, and for this reason they are called the functional psychoses. They include schizophrenia and the two main forms of depression, namely endogenous or unipolar depression and manic-depressive psychosis or bipolar depression.

Pain other than that arising from the disease giving rise to the condition is not found as a symptom in the organic psychoses. However, it does occur in a small number of patients with depressive psychosis though rarely in hypomania or schizophrenia.

ANXIETY NEUROSIS AND PAIN

Anxiety is a universal experience and, although essential to some extent for normal mental life, it may give rise to a great deal of distress if excessive and prolonged. Proneness to develop anxiety to stresses in the environment is a lifelong personality trait in those susceptible and the range of circumstances giving rise to it vary enormously. It is an experience which occurs not only in 'pure culture' as an anxiety neurosis, or anxiety reaction, but in other disorders too. These include other neuroses, for example obsessional and hysterical neurosis and also the psychoses, alcoholism and early dementia. When anxiety occurs as part of a tendency to respond to a wide range of stresses in the environment it is termed 'free floating' but when attached to a specific fear, for example of animals or insects, heights or open spaces, it forms an integral part of a phobia. The latter is fear which is out of proportion to the threat of the stimulus causing it as in the case of a fear of spiders or butterflies, and when it incapacitates an individual socially it becomes the basis of a phobic anxiety neurosis.

An anxiety neurosis is a state in which excessive and ill-founded anxiety occurs amounting to acute fear and panic at times. Somatic symptoms due to alterations in the activity of the autonomic nervous system and less often of endocrine activity are present and the changes in the individual's emotional and physical state have secondary effects upon intellectual activities, including concentration, memory and judgement. Anxiety reactions are very common but vary in form with some patients complaining chiefly of emotional discomforts, whereas others are concerned mostly about physical changes. The former describe feelings of being 'tense', 'strung up' or 'on edge', all expressions which give the sense of tension. Complaints of excessive anxiety, constant nervousness and being panicky at times are common and those who experience tachycardia, excessive sweating, dryness of the mouth and tremulousness, may interpret their physical feelings in more general terms, such as having 'butterflies in the stomach', shortness of breath which when severe amounts to choking and, at times, feelings of imminent collapse or even death. The anxious person is restless, unable to sit still for any length of time and may fidget ceaselessly. In less acute phases patients' complaints are of tiredness, loss of energy and insomnia, together with alteration in eating habits which may include increased or reduced consumption of food. There are usually difficulties in getting to sleep with initial sleeplessness and later restlessness and frequent sudden wakening.

Complaints of pain are common both in the constitutionally anxious person and one who has a fully developed anxiety neurosis. Most complaints are related to the head, face, neck, chest or muscles of the limbs. Headaches are described as 'tight bands', a 'weight on the head', or even 'explosions inside the skull'. Electrophysiological studies reveal evidence of increased tension in scalp, facial and cervical muscles, which accounts for the complaints of pain. Similar findings have been made in lumbar and limb muscles too. These are part of a wider range of physiological disturbances and all may occur intermittently in association with the fluctuations in the subjective sense of anxiety. Palpation of larger muscle groups, for example in the lumbar and cervical regions when pain is present reveals that they are in spasm, tender to the touch and that movement of that part of the body is not only limited but associated with increased pain on attempts to provoke movement. In some areas known as trigger spots there are exquisitely tender nodules which when pressed give rise to locally acute pain and more widespread pain too. Usually the patient's history and emotional state are sufficient to explain the presence of pain due to muscle spasm, but it must always be remembered that to reach a diagnosis of 'psychogenic pain' a reasonable search for organic causes has to be made because in a number of instances there may be a physical lesion which in an anxiety-prone person is producing a reactive and intense emotional disturbance. Attention to the patient's attitudes to symptoms seems important for it might be expected that the individual with an organic disorder would be more preoccupied with the question of the cause of the pain than somebody with anxiety arising for other reasons, although this is not always the case.

DEPRESSION AND PAIN

When occurring as a response to an identifiable stress within the environment, say bereavement or other form of loss, and when the sufferer retains contact with the reality of the surrounding world and is not troubled by delusions or hallucinations, depression is regarded as neurotic. It is differentiated from severe depressive illness with psychotic features and from manic-depressive psychosis. A depressive neurosis is expressed in changes of mood, intellect and physical health. The depressed person is filled with misery, the depth of which may be sharpened by any contact with thoughts of the factors causing it, worsening when the individual is alone and lessening when in the company of others, or in situations which give rise to distraction. There is a sense of loss, of joy having gone out of life, and there are feelings of hopelessness and pessimism about the future. Levels of energy and interest fall, concentration, memory and judgement deteriorate, and physical symptoms of various kinds may appear. Appetite changes are common, sometimes with over-eating and a marked increase in weight, and sometimes almost with total loss of appetite and weight loss. Sleep is slow to come and the night is troubled by dreams with a noticeably depressive content and periods of wakefulness. Psychotic depressive disorders differ in that there is less often an obvious precipitating factor, the level of depression is more constant and is not relieved by changes in circumstances, it tends to be more pronounced in the early part of the day. It is often associated with delusions which are unassailably held false beliefs that the individual is doomed, that he is poor or that he has been the cause of distress to others, and so forth. In some cases the depression is associated with extreme restlessness and agitation, and in others with apathy, which at times leads into a situation of complete immobility or depressive stupor. In psychotic depressions appetite is lost and there may be a very rapid reduction of weight. There is also loss of libido and the individual may view the future with such foreboding and his circumstances with such misery that suicide is attempted, perhaps successfully.

Complaints of aches and pains are common in depressive disorders of the reactive type and are associated with a tendency to develop hypochondriasis as part of physical illness. Pain is a much less common complaint in patients with severe or endogenous depression but when it occurs it is also associated with hypochondriacal preoccupation and, although it is uncertain why this should be so, it is said that the development of physical symptoms is an unconsciously operating mechanism whereby attention is turned away from intolerable mental suffering to physical suffering which, though considerable at times, is coped with more easily. If the process is completely successful the patient does not appear to be depressed and the depression is said to be masked but, when incomplete, 'mental pain' or depression, and physical pain coexist. An alternative biological explanation is that the neurochemical systems subserving both pain modulation and mood overlap. Therefore, an abnormality in these systems may well alter mood and simultaneously lead to the experience of pain. The latter often occurs at the site of previous tissue injury, perhaps because once injured any part of the body gives rise to abnormal neuronal activity which, however, does not enter consciousness and give rise to the experience of pain unless there is a fault in the modulating mechanism. The key neurotransmitter in this sequence of events appears to be serotonin and antidepressant drugs which increase the availability of this substance in the central nervous system often relieve co-existing pain and depression. As mentioned in an earlier chapter the tendency to develop pain in the face of life's difficulties is characteristic of the 'pain-prone person', though depressive illness with pain develops in others who do not have the hallmarks of this particular personality type. The site of pain in depressive disorders varies but, as in anxiety states, headache and facial pains are common, and so too is lumbar and abdominal pain. All have marked psychological characteristics and, although the patient complains to the doctor of pain, depression is mentioned but generally it is seen by both as the consequence of the pain and concern about health.

A rare but important example of complete masking of depression is that in which patients experience intractable, dull facial pain which is felt deeply, poorly localised and which sometimes crosses the midline. Typical depressive symptoms are not expressed but patients complain chiefly of lethargy, fatigue and tension with disorders of sleep as well as pain. By nature the individual tends to have an obsessional personality, being over-conscientious and meticulous in everyday life. Where the history of the condition is short, that is a matter of months only, response to antidepressant drugs is good, but where it has been present for several years and there have been surgical treatments by dentists or surgeons the outlook is poor.

A careful history should place the various symptoms in depressive disorders with pain in perspective against the background of possible stressful circumstances, and successful treatment of depression, which also relieves pain, confirms the diagnosis of a depressive illness. It is worth remembering that when chronic pain clearly precedes the onset of depression by many weeks, months, or even years, the change in mental state is likely to be a reaction to prolonged suffering. In contrast, when the onset of pain and depression appear to coincide, and especially when there is little or no evidence of a physical basis for pain and events which have a strong emotional content have occurred, pain is probably part of a disorder of mood.

HYPOCHONDRIASIS AND PAIN

A hypochondriacal neurosis is defined as a condition in which excessive and morbid concern with health in general, or some particular aspect of physical or mental health predominates. It is important to see hypochondriasis in a broader context, as an attitude towards health which is characterised by its close association with emotional tension and a need to discuss the concerns felt with others, whether they are family, friends or doctors. Hypochondriasis is one of the common problems of medical practice as about 10 per cent of all regular attenders at general practitioners' surgeries have hypochondriacal tendencies in one form or another. Concern about health varies from a personality trait which may present as excessive absorption with physical fitness, or with the functioning of some particular part of the body such as the bowels, with the unnecessary consumption of patent remedies, an aspect of human behaviour which attracts a very high level of exploitation by commercial concerns, to a serious mental illness in which there is an incontravertible belief that part of the body is seriously affected by disease against all evidence to the contrary.

In summary, the elements, one or more of which seem basic to the concept of hypochondriasis are:

1. A preoccupation with bodily functions.
2. A fear of disease.
3. An unshakeable belief in the existence of serious disease for which there is no foundation in reality.

Although hypochondriasis does occur in the absence of any other symptoms it is far more commonly found as a secondary feature of a neurosis or a psychotic illness. In anxiety neurosis excessive preoccupation with the physiological sequelae of anxiety and, in phobic states fear of cancer, heart disease or venereal disease may be the centre of concern. In all forms of depressive illness hypochondriasis may become so prominent as to mask the depression. Hysteria and hypochondriasis may be difficult to distinguish at times, but this can be achieved by careful analysis of the patient's previous personality, the history of his or her condition and current mental and physical state. Hypochondriacal symptoms also occur in schizophrenia and at the onset of physical disorders in later life which lead to dementia.

Hypochondriacal patients are more likely than others to have had previous symptoms of physical illness. Their illnesses seem to be more like those suffered by their mothers than is the case with non-hypochondriacal individuals suggesting that early learning about illness and attitudes to it, especially over-solicitousness at the times of ill health from an otherwise emotionally detached mother, can be important in the development of a health conscious personality. They have also been shown to have poorer marital and social adjustments. Hypochondriacal symptoms appear most often in middle age, perhaps because of the occurence at that time of life of the early changes of physical decline, the appearance with increasing frequency of disease in the individual's associates, family and friends and the realisation that peaks of attainment once sought have either been reached or past with former goals becoming unattainable. The reaction to the disappointments, frustrations and failures takes one of a number of forms with depression and hypochondriasis being the most common.

Hypochondriacal symptoms centre upon disorders in the head, face, neck, abdomen and chest, in order of preference and they are based upon the musculoskeletal, gastro-intestinal and nervous systems. Complaints of pain are very common, occurring in approximately three quarters of those regarded as having hypochondriacal symptoms with headache, facial pains, chest, low back pains and vague limb pains in order of frequency. Amongst children complaints of abdominal pain without evidence of physical abnormality are very common, though whether they are truly hypochondriacal or rather to be regarded as expressions of distress arising out of difficulties in relationships with others, as is usually the case and as such are depressive or hysterical conversion symptoms, is uncertain.

Physical examination of the patient with hypochondriacal symptoms generally reveals little or no evidence of physical abnormalities, although certain individuals do over-react to minor physical disorders and are regarded as having hypochondriacal personality traits which lead to exaggeration of trivial disturbances of physical function (see page 47).

Persistent complaints of pain, or other hypochondriacal symptoms when associated with a depressive psychosis or schizophrenia are likely to disappear with successful treatment of the primary condition. Where hypochondriasis is present as part of a disorder of personality development the symptoms are likely to be much more resistant to treatment.

HYSTERIA AND PAIN

In any discussion of hysteria care must be taken not to confuse the reactions of an individual with an hysterical personality (see page 46) and an hysterical neurosis (i.e. an hysterical conversion disorder).

An hysterical neurosis is one in which the symptoms have the function of reducing excessive levels of emotion and where the individual concerned is unaware of the connection between physical symptoms and underlying conflicts. In other words there is dissociation of the physical from the psychological elements of the disorder. The physical symptoms, known as conversion phenomena, which may occur include changes in consciousness with prolonged periods of memory loss (hysterical amnesia), paralysis and sensory loss in the limbs, paralysis of bladder function, aphonia, blindness, deafness or seizures. Psychogenic pain is frequently regarded as a conversion symptom and as with other symptoms in an hysterical neurosis it is unassociated with an adequate organic cause and there is, on careful examination of the patient's history, evidence of psychological precipitants. Hysterical conversion symptoms do arise from time to time in association with organic disease, following surgical operations, or even diagnostic manipulations, such as lumbar puncture, dilatation and curettage of the cervix, laryngoscopy, and others. They do not occur with greater frequency in any particular personality type and are the result of the individual facing an overwhelming psychological stress. For example, hysterical blindness may occur in soldiers for whom removal from the battlefield reduces or removes the prospect of imminent death or severe disablement.

The unconscious mental defence mechanism of dissociation which leads to the production of physical disability produces an important gain (primary gain) for the patient by preventing potentially harmful levels of emotion reaching consciousness. The disability may then produce its own advantages (secondary gains) of which the patient is often aware and these include increased concern by others for the sufferer, liberation from responsibility and, nowadays, the prospect of financial support by the State. The striking feature of patients with hysterical neurosis is the discrepancy between the severity of their disability and the level of concern they appear to show. This contrasts with normal individuals who when stricken with sudden blindness, paralysis or severe pain, exhibit marked anxiety and concern about the cause of their problem, seeking relief as rapidly as possible. However, despite the low level of concern shown, the patient with hysterical conversion symptoms is insistent that his problems are physical and not emotional as a continued defence against exposure to underlying psychological difficulties. Most reject the suggestion of psychiatric help, at least initially, and tacit acceptance that the symptom may not be physical in origin or permanent is usually the first step in a successful treatment programme.

One of the main stumbling blocks preventing a doctor reaching this point with his patient is the emphasis placed upon reaching a diagnosis of hysteria solely by excluding physical causes for the disability. During this process the patient gradually forms the opinion that doctors believe there is nothing wrong and that pain is imaginary. A doctor must accept that the patient's report of the experiences of the illness are true and that pain is present or the symptoms are genuine, although all his instincts founded in long experience of pain arising from physical causes lead him to believe otherwise. During history-taking patients often give clear indications that others do not appreciate the level of their suffering, or that they do nothing to help recovery. At times they show hostility and resentment towards doctors who have examined and treated them believing that they have caused harm, which may indeed be true. All are signs that the patient feels rejected and that perhaps others regard him or her as weak and worthless. However, at times the opposite emotion is expressed and the patient expresses overwhelming thanks to a doctor who has been totally unable to provide a solution to the physical problem but who has expressed a positive wish to help at a level of understanding that is comforting and reassuring.

Malingering

It has been said that 'nothing resembles malingering more than hysteria, and nothing resembles hysteria more than malingering'. Herein lies one of the conundrums of life in surgical, medical, and psychiatric practice. However, there are several clues which make the wary clinician suspect malingering—a state in which an individual consciously and deliberately falsifies physical symptoms, including pain. First, in civil life, the main motive for deceit is centred upon complaints of a physical nature in relation to an accident for which compensation is sought. Only rarely does it involve the avoidance of difficult and dangerous work, although this is an important reason amongst Servicemen. Clinical examination may reveal some form of abnormality but it will either be very slight in comparison with the level of disability of which the individual complains, or patently be manufactured. Pain is an ideal symptom as it is difficult to assess, or disprove, and investigation will often reveal that, apparently, the disorder, though longlasting, appears to be unchanging. But, careful observation of the patient by a doctor, relatives or friends, may reveal that behaviour is normal when the patient thinks he is alone. Further investigation may uncover a premorbid history of similar events of dishonesty and of difficult family problems, especially financial ones. Although the patient does not work, often he has not given up his pleasures in life. He may well be unwilling to submit to hospitalisation, or surgery, and is likely to default on any treatment given. Offers of employment are usually refused, even though they may involve the use of what might be regarded as residual and available skills. For obvious reasons treatment is difficult but its essence lies in uncovering the deceit leaving the patient with the certain knowledge that his false symptoms have been recognised. If this goal is achieved the patient tends to discontinue attendance at the clinic or surgery and, after a suitable interval, he may also recover!

PAIN AND SCHIZOPHRENIA

The term schizophrenia covers a group of psychoses, that is, disorders in which there is a fundamental disturbance of personality, a characteristic distortion of thinking, often a sense of being controlled by alien forces, delusions (false beliefs held with conviction and which are out of context with the individual's culture), disturbed perception, abnormal mood, and withdrawal. Nevertheless, clear consciousness and intellectual capacity are usually maintained.

The disturbances described occur in different combinations and these, taken into consideration with other factors such as family history and individual's personality development, have led to the identification of several forms of schizophrenia. These are:

1. Simple schizophrenia
2. Hebephrenic schizophrenia
3. Catatonic schizophrenia
4. Paranoid schizophrenia

Of these the only one in which pain is likely to occur as part of the symptoms is hebephrenia.

Hebephrenia is a disorder which makes its appearance in adolescence or early adult life (*hebe*, Greek, 'youth'). The appearance of obvious symptoms may be preceded by a period during which the individual withdraws increasingly into his or her own private world, shunning others and spending long periods alone. Interests in mysticism, magic, philosophy or more vague subjects such as the meaning of life and the cosmos, may be expressed. Later, changes in mood become prominent with the sudden appearance of episodes of depression, or at times euphoria, though generally the individual's emotions are shallow and inappropriate. Thoughts are disorganised to a variable extent and disordered perception takes the form of delusions and hallucinations which, however, are not always present. Sometimes there are hypochondriacal complaints, or even feelings that the body is changing. With regard to the latter, changes of sex are sometimes felt to be occuring. Included amongst the hypochondriacal complaints are those of pain, which is usually ill-defined, and at times described in bizarre terms. Behaviour is unpredictable, and strange and repetitive movements of the face or limbs may occur. The individual may smile secretly, at times giggling or grimacing without obvious cause.

Clearly pain occuring in hebephrenic schizophrenia is unlikely to be diagnosed as anything other than part of that condition if it has the characteristics of 'psychogenic pain'. But, it should be remembered that however severe a mental illness may be patients also develop physical disorders from time to time. If this occurs when the schizophrenic illness is florid, distortion of complaints about pain may be misunderstood and the doctor must be more than usually careful in his questioning of the patient and physical examination.

PAIN AND MENTAL SUBNORMALITY

Mental subnormality, characterised by 'a state of arrested or incomplete development of mind', is defined arbitarily in terms of levels of intelligence. Mentally handicapped individuals have an intelligence quotient of 85 or less with a mean level for the population being 100. If the I.Q. lies between 68 and 85 the person may well lead an independent life in the community, but when below this increasing amounts of support, care and protection are required. An I.Q. of 36 to 51 is regarded as a moderate degree of retardation, between 20 and 35 severe retardation, and below this profound retardation. Contrary to popular opinion reactivity to artificially induced noxious stimuli amongst mentally subnormal individuals does not differ from that exhibited by normal people, except at the profoundly retarded level. In other words, ability to experience pain is not related to intelligence except when it is very low indeed and the main problem faced by the doctor dealing with the handicapped is their lack of sophistication in communication and ability to communicate their experiences to any but those who understand them well through long and close contact. Therefore, evaluation of the subnormal individual's physical state depends heavily on careful physical examination and evaluation of behaviour using the knowledge others have of the sufferer's change in his or her physical and emotional state. Confusion in diagnosis may occur because a number of severely and profoundly subnormal people mutilate themselves quite badly at times and, as they do not appear to experience pain in proportion to the severity of the mutilation, the view that they cannot experience pain may be established erroneously.

PART THREE

Physical and psychological methods of relieving pain

13

General aspects of pain relief

The effective treatment of pain depends upon careful evaluation and application of the appropriate techniques of management to it. Evaluation involves taking the patient's history, paying particular attention to the cause of pain, an accurate assessment of its severity at the time of examination and in terms of its hourly and daily variations, and the influence of personal and environment factors upon it. This should be followed by a careful physical examination with concentration upon the affected part of the body. All too often, because of lack of time, lack of interest or even lack of knowledge, these simple steps are not followed resulting in an inaccurate assessment which leads to mistakes in later care. Pain due to trauma, acute physical illness or following surgery, is easily linked to its source, but, perhaps, because interest lies chiefly in other areas, attention to pain relief is rather neglected by doctors and nurses alike. Many individuals, including members of the medical profession, can testify to the inadequate treatment of their own post-operative pain and it is not unknown for them to 'smuggle' their own supplies of analgesic drugs into hospital and for their non-medical fellows to take the precaution of hoarding drugs for later pain relief.

In chronic illness treatment of pain should be effective as there is greater time for assessment and for trials of treatments in a search for the most satisfactory form of pain relief. Regrettably there is evidence that control of pain in these circumstances also leaves much to be desired and the main sources of difficulty appear to be failure to appreciate the very important role of emotional and social factors in the patient's behaviour and level of pain, and failure to use appropriate forms of physical treatment, particularly the inappropriate use of analgesic drugs. When unable to find convincing evidence of an organic source for pain a whole series of difficulties arise. However, the doctor should not proceed to carry out numerous, irrelevant and perhaps dangerous investigations merely for the sake 'of completeness', but on the other hand should not dismiss the patient as 'neurotic or hysterical' as sometimes happens. Instead he or she should take a more careful history, seeking evidence of emotional difficulties which may be giving rise to pain or at least accentuating its severity and complaints about it and if necessary refer the patient either to a doctor skilled in the treatment of pain problems, or to a clinic in which doctors with a common interest in pain but from different specialties in medicine gather.

Management of pain is the course of action taken to provide relief and is based upon two approaches to the symptoms. First, attention to the sufferer's general comfort and wellbeing, and second upon the use of specific pain relieving measures. The former include removal of causes of pain, the use of rest, or judicious amounts of exercise where appropriate, and the relief of emotional tension, for example anxiety about the physical and social aspects of the illness. They also include relief of other symptoms which are distressing, such as diarrhoea, vomiting or breathlessness. The range of measures for pain relief is wide, varying from simple ones like the application of heat, the use of splinting to prevent movement, and the use of specific pain-relieving substances, including analgesic drugs, antispasmodics and antacids, to the use of more specialised methods which are based on techniques used by surgeons, anaesthetists or pyschiatrist. The possibility of using methods of treatment regarded as less conventional and practised within and outside these specialties should be considered on appropriate occasions. Chief amongst them are acupuncture, hypnotherapy and relaxation, and they, together with other methods are described in this section.

GENERAL MEASURES FOR PAIN RELIEF

The value of rest, which means relief gained by reduction in work either of the whole person or part of his body, is considerable in pain relief; a fact that has been known for many centuries and a subject which forms the main theme of an early and well known text by a London surgeon, John Hilton, entitled *Lectures on Rest and Pain* and first published in 1863. Rest may be regarded as relief for the individual from either physical or emotional stresses that promote or exaggerate pain. For example, time away from work either as a deliberate therapeutic manoeuvre which is frequently used by doctors to facilitate healing of wounds and infections in a wide variety of disorders, or in the form of a holiday specifically designed to bring relief from the mental pressures of work or other stressful aspects of everyday life. Hilton commented upon this use of rest and also upon the more specific attempts to rest particular areas or organs of the body affected by disease or injury, or the use of drugs to give ease to those in mental turmoil. For example, splinting of fractured limbs does not merely keep the bones in good alignment but also prevents movement which helps the healing process and reduces pain. A cervical collar is commonly used in the treatment of spondylosis and by preventing excessive movements of the neck helps to reduce reflex muscle spasm and therefore pain. A similar effect is gained by the wearing of a lumbar support where back pain is due to reflex muscle spasm in lumbar disc disease. Rest can be brought about by surgical operations too in which inflamed regions of the body have been temporarily removed from their normal activities, for example where a temporary colostomy is used in cases of pelvic abscess secondary to diverticular disease of the large bowel, or where an anastomosis between the stomach and small bowel is performed to divert gastric contents from an inflamed and ulcerated duodenum. There are many other examples where either man or nature induces rest in this way, and the principle of its use will be clear on consideration of the examples given.

The value of heat for pain relief is well established and achieves its effect in three ways. First, it gives a feeling of comfort leading to relaxation, next it has a specific effect on increasing local blood supply thereby increasing local blood flow, reducing the pain producing metabolites, and last it may act as a 'counter irritant' which means that the heat, if sufficient, causes pain relief by strongly stimulating the skin which in turn leads to the operation of pain modulating mechanisms in the central nervous system. Rubifacients, that is compounds designed to cause mild irritation of the skin when massaged into it, act in a similar manner. Heat may be applied locally, often in the form of a hot water bottle, or may be given as radiant heat (infra-red radiation) as is common practice in departments of physiotherapy where it is used to treat musculoskeletal pain. Similar effects may be gained by massage using 'rubbing oils' which are firm favourites with athletes. Probably these act primarily as lubricants with the massage itself providing the relief by increasing muscle blood flow and reduced emotional tension.

14

Analgesic drugs for pain relief

Pain relief may be gained by using drugs which act upon the nervous system by affecting perceptual mechanisms and the emotional response to pain as in the case of narcotic drugs. It may be gained by interfering with the metabolism of peripheral pain-producing substances in the tissues, such as the kinins and prostaglandins, as happens when antipyretic drugs and those which improve blood flow to ischaemic areas (vasodilators) are used, or when irritant substances, such as hydrochloric acid in the stomach, are neutralised.

ANALGESICS

Analgesics abolish or reduce pain without causing loss of consciousness in contrast to general anaesthetics which do both. If one could manufacture the ideal analgesic it would have the following properties:

1. Reduce early perception of pain.
2. Produce analgesia over a wide range of pain levels.
3. Act satisfactorily whether given by mouth or parenterally.
4. Be effective at all ages and in all disorders which give rise to pain.
5. Produce few and minor side effects.
6. Be free from any tendency to produce tolerance and drug dependence.

Unfortunately the endless search for such a drug has not yet revealed the perfect analgesic but we do have access to a wide range of compounds which vary in their potency and mode of action thereby giving a useful pharmacological battery with which to relieve pain. The main classes of analgesics are shown in Table 12.

NARCOTIC ANALGESICS

The narcotic analgesics (narkosis, Greek, 'a benumbing') produce

Table 12 Classification of analgesic drugs

Narcotic analgesics	
1. Alkaloids of opium:	morphine, codeine papaveretum
2. Semisynthetic alkaloids:	diamorphine, dihydrocodeine
3. Thebaine derivatives:	buprenorphine
4. Synthetic drugs with a morphine-like action:	levorphanol, pethidine phenoperidine, fentanyl, oxycodone
5. Benzomorphan derivatives:	pentazocine, ethoheptazine
6. Methadone group:	methadone, dipipanone, dextromoramide, dextropropoxyphene
Antipyretic analgesics and anti-inflammatory drugs	
1. Salicylates:	aspirin
2. Compounds related to salicylates:	mefenamic acid, flufenamic acid
3. Analine derivatives:	diflunisal, paracetamol
4. Indole derivatives:	indomethacin
5. Pyrazoline derivatives:	phenylbutazone oxyphenbutazone

analgesia and depress activity of the nervous system by acting centrally by contrast with the milder antipyretic analgesics which act more peripherally in the relief of pain. They are used to relieve severe pain having the added valuable property of producing mental tranquillity or euphoria in the case of the most potent members, though unfortunately this is linked with their tendency to produce mental and sometimes physical dependence upon the drug.

Derivatives of opium

For centuries opium, a drug extracted from the dried juice of the unripe capsule of the opium poppy (*papaver somniferum*) was used in pain relief, and in some cultures socially for the production of euphoria. Crude opium contains two active constituents, the phenanthrene and the isoquinoline derivatives. From the former morphine, codeine and thebaine are derived, and from the latter papaverine and narcotine.

Morphine

Morphine (Morpheus, god of dreams) is an alkaloid derived from opium and is the most commonly used powerful analgesic drug. As such it is the standard agent against which the efficacy of other compounds is assessed. Morphine has been in use as opium (from the Greek for 'juice') for more than 2000 years and an eloquent testimony to its value was given by the famous 17th century English physician, Dr Thomas Sydenham, who wrote, 'Among the remedies which it has pleased Almighty God to give man to relieve his sufferings, none is so universal and so efficacious as opium'. Also, he introduced tincture of opium, known as Laudanum, into medicine—a preparation which was freely available at one time and, due to public abuse, the cause of much misery as a result of its addictive properties. For an enlightened account of the problem of addiction to Laudanum the reader should consult 'Confessions of an English Opium Eater' by Thomas de Quincey (1785–1859) who began taking the drug when an undergraduate at Oxford University.

Morphine exerts a pain relieving action centrally, perhaps by inhibiting the release of transmitter substances in the brain, such as acetylcholine. It is known to suppress the activity of connections between the frontal lobes and the thalamus in the same way as alcohol and by this means reduces anxiety and promotes euphoria, a property which is used in the control of severe pain and to reduce anxiety in conditions of shock. Furthermore, morphine raises the threshold for the appreciation of pain and induces sleep. Morphine also interrupts neurotransmission in the spinal cord by blocking afferent nerve input in the dorsal horn region. It causes depression of the respiratory centre by reducing sensitivity to raised levels of carbon dioxide in the blood and it suppresses the cough reflex, a property of this group of drugs widely used in medical practice. Care is required when using morphine in situations where respiratory depression could be hazardous, for example in patients with pulmonary diseases, or women in labour where passage of the drug across the placenta will depress the respiratory centres in the brain of the unborn or newly born child. However, under other circumstances the pain relieving properties of morphine far outweigh its effects on respiration. For example, severe pain from an upper abdominal wound may lead to more pulmonary complications by causing gross reduction of movements of the chest wall than morphine, which paradoxically improves respiratory activity by eliminating, or greatly reducing, pain and anxiety.

Unfortunately morphine also has excitatory effects upon the central nervous system which produce unpleasant effects including nausea and vomiting due to stimulation of the medullary emetic centre and vestibular apparatus. It reduces the tone and mobility of smooth muscle which in some circumstances may cause difficulties such as constipation, but then again this property is of value in the control of diarrhoea. By contrast it causes contraction of the smooth muscle of the sphincter of Oddi at the junction between the common bile duct and duodenum, thus leading to worsening of symptoms of biliary obstruction giving rise to colic if given in this condition.

The depressant action of morphine and similar drugs such as pethidine can be countered where undue respiratory depression has occurred by using specific antagonists. The drug of choice for the reversal of the effect of morphine is naloxone (N-allylnoroxymorphine) because unlike other antagonists it is pure in its action, lacking any of the effects of morphine itself. It will also antagonise the effects of pentazocine.

It should be remembered that in cases of morphine addiction administration of an antagonist will induce withdrawal symptoms. The usual dose of morphine sulphate by injection for an adult is 10 to 20 mg given subcutaneously. Care should be taken where the patient shows evidence of circulatory failure as distribution of drug from the injection site may be delayed with the result that further doses give rise to undesirable toxicity due to accumulation of the unmetabolised drug. In the treatment of chronic pain in patients with malignant diseases it is preferable to prescribe oral morphine if possible and the dose regime, which is very flexible, ranges from 10 mg to a maximum of 90 mg several times each day, (see pp. 216 and 219).

Morphine forms 50 per cent of the compound papaveretum which also contains very small amounts of papaverine, codeine and narcotine. A 20 mg dose of papaveretum (Omnopon) is used in combination with 0.4 mg of hyoscine (Scopolamine) by intramuscular injection as a premedication for surgery. The last named drug causes sedation and mild amnesia.

Morphine derivatives

In an attempt to avoid the problems associated with the use of morphine, especially lowering of consciousness and the development of tolerance and addiction, extensive research has been carried out into the properties of compounds derived from it. As yet no better successor has been discovered, but nevertheless there are a number of useful analgesics which come from this source and which are in daily use.

Diamorphine hydrochloride (Heroin)

This drug is a semi-synthetic derivative of morphine and more powerful than its parent compound, having an analgesic effect which appears more rapidly but which lasts for a shorter period of time. It causes greater respiratory depression but less nausea than morphine and also produces vomiting, constipation and marked sedation. It is very likely to cause drug dependence and for this reason its use in Britain is strictly controlled and forbidden in the United States.

The dose for adults is 5 to 10 mg given by subcutaneous injection and it is chiefly used to control pain in terminal malignancy and attacks of myocardial infarction in which situation it is the drug of choice. As diamorphine in solution breaks down quite quickly into monoacetylmorphine and morphine, it should be prepared freshly for each injection from the chemically stable powder form.

Dihydrocodeine (DF 118)

This is a semi-synthetic derivative of codeine and is intermediate in its analgesic effects between the latter and morphine. It is used to control moderate to severe pain and its side effects, which sometimes make it intolerable to patients, include dizziness and nausea. Habituation to the drug occurs and therefore it should be prescribed only for short periods, say four to six weeks, and its effects should be checked regularly by the doctor. Like morphine, dihydrocodeine may be given as an oral preparation to patients with severe pain due to malignant diseases, (see pp. 216 and 219). It is administered in doses of 30 to 60 mg by mouth or 50 mg by intramuscular injection.

Codeine phosphate

This drug has about one-tenth the potency of morphine but it is stronger than the antipyretic analgesics. It is used to control mild to moderate pain, diarrhoea and cough. The common commercial practice of combining it with other analgesics almost certainly reduces its potency. For example, tablets including codeine with aspirin, or paracetamol are freely available. Codeine phosphate tablets are given to adults in doses ranging from 15 to 60 mg.

Buprenorphine (Temgesic)

Buprenorphine is a potent long-acting analgesic derived from thebaine and structurally related to morphine. It is 35 times more potent than morphine and its analgesic action lasts up to 10 hours. Its side-effects are similar to, but less marked than, those of morphine and the risk of dependence is lower. The commonest side-effects are drowsiness, respiratory depression, nausea, dizziness and sweating. The drug is used to control post-operative pain and also in the treatment of chronic pain due to cancer. It is useful for the control of pain at night because of its duration of action and, if it is desirable to avoid injection, the drug may be given in a dose of 0.4 mg three times daily as tablets to be dissolved under the tongue. When given by injection doses of 0.2 to 0.4 mg are given three times a day.

SYNTHETIC DRUGS WHICH RESEMBLE MORPHINE IN THEIR EFFECT

Pethidine

This drug is unrelated chemically to morphine and was discovered in the search for compounds with atropine-like properties needed to reduce muscle spasm, but was found to be a powerful analgesic one-eighth to one-tenth the potency of morphine. Onset of analgesia is comparable with morphine taking only minutes to appear, and lasting two to three hours if given by intramuscular injection. It is less effective when given by mouth. In equivalent doses to morphine it produces respiratory depression and because of its atropine-like properties causes hypotension, tachycardia and dryness of the mouth. Nausea and vomiting are less common than with morphine and its side-effects can be reversed by morphine antagonists, for example nalorphine. Apart from simple analgesia it is used specifically to abolish smooth muscle spasm and is of great value in treating ureteric colic, and other painful intestinal disorders. It is also used extensively in obstetrics because it causes increased uterine activity and relaxation of spasm of the muscles of the cervix. In combination with drugs of the phenothiazine group, for example chlorpromazine, it provides good premedication for minor surgical procedures where full anaesthesia is not required. It is important to remember that pethidine must not be given where psychotropic drugs of the monoamine oxidase inhibitor group are being taken as this is likely to precipitate excitement and/or a hypertensive crisis perhaps with coma, hypotension or even death (see page 172). Pethidine is a drug to which tolerance develops quickly and which induces dependency. It is given in doses of 50 to 100 mg by intramuscular injection in adults, and a dose between 75 and 100 mg is equal in potency to 10 mg of morphine sulphate.

PIPERIDINE DERIVATIVES OF PETHIDINE

Phenoperidine and fentanyl (Operidine and Sublimaze)

These drugs, which are chemically related to pethidine but are much more potent, are used in anaesthetic practice to produce analgesia. Both cause marked respiratory depression and they are given only under strictly controlled conditions by anaesthetists. A combination of fentanyl 0.5 mg and droperidol 2.5 mg/ml (Thalamonal) is used to produce neuroleptanalgesia, which means that for a short period of 30 to 60 minutes patients experience profound analgesia with mental detachment of such a degree that minor surgery or investigations, such as the performance of cardiac catheterisation, can be carried out with ease in both adults and young children.

Phenoperidine and fentanyl should not be given within 14 days of the administration of a monoamine oxidase inhibitor.

Oxycodone pectinate (Proladone)
This is a valuable and potent analgesic drug which is particularly useful because it gives prolonged analgesia of 8 to 14 hours with less sedation than morphine. It can be given to cover the night hours and is administered by suppository in a dose of 30 mg.

Levorphanol tartrate (Dromoran)
This is a drug similar in potency to morphine in terms of its analgesic properties. It is not a powerful anxiolytic and is less likely to produce vomiting though, as in the case of morphine, there is a risk of habituation. As it is less prone to produce vomiting it is used in ambulant patients with moderate to severe pain and is given in a dose of 1 to 5 mg by injection or, because it is one of the most efficient and long-acting oral narcotics, by mouth in a dose of 1.5 to 4.5 mg once or twice daily.

BENZOMORPHAN DERIVATIVES

Pentazocine (Fortral)
This drug is a weak narcotic antagonist. In other words it can block the action of morphine by competition for receptor sites in the brain which means also that if given to a morphine addict it will produce withdrawal symptoms. The drug produces analgesia without marked sedation, respiratory depression or euphoria. Its side effects include mild respiratory depression, nausea, vomiting, dizziness and hallucinations, though none of these, with the exception of nausea and dizziness, are common if the lower doses are used. The drug is not regarded as one which produces physical or emotional dependence, though cases of this have been recorded.

The potency of pentazocine at a dose of 30 mg by intramuscular injection is equal to 10 mg of morphine and it is normally given to adults in doses of 30 mg by intramuscular injection, or 50 mg by mouth for moderate pain. It is also available in suppository form, (50 mg).

Ethoheptazine citrate
This drug is a weak analgesic with some antispasmodic effects and therefore it is of use in painful musculoskeletal disorders. It is given

in tablet form in a dose of 75 to 150 mg three to four times daily, in combination with either aspirin (Zactrin) or with paracetamol (Zactipar). It is not a drug of habituation.

THE METHADONE GROUP

Methadone (Physeptone)
This drug is not closely related to morphine but produces similar analgesic and respiratory effects. It may also produce dizziness, nausea and a dry mouth in ambulatory patients, but has the advantage of good absorption when taken by mouth. It does not produce sedation. Dependence can occur, but nevertheless its chief use is in the treatment of morphine addiction. The dose of this drug when given for the relief of severe pain is 5 to 10 mg three or four times each day either by mouth or by intramuscular injection.

Dipipanone (with cyclizene; Diconal).
This drug is related chemically to methadone and has similar properties both with regard to its efficacy and toxicity. It is commonly given for the relief of moderate to severe pain, usually in an oral dose of 10 mg in combination with cyclizene in a dose of 30 mg. It may be given subcutaneously or intramuscularly in a dose of 25 to 50 mg.

Dextromoramide (Palfium)
This drug is also chemically related to methadone and similar in properties to it and dipipanone. It is given for the relief of moderate to severe pain in a dose of 5 to 20 mg three or four times each day by mouth or by intramuscular injection.

Dextropropoxyphene hydrochloride (with Paracetamol, Distalgesic)
The potency of this drug is comparable with codeine, but unlike the latter does not suppress cough. It is well absorbed when taken by mouth and does not cause habituation. It is available in tablet form in combination with 325 mg of paracetamol and the adult dose is 65 mg when taken by mouth (2 tablets).

ANTIPYRETIC ANALGESICS AND ANTI-INFLAMMATORY AGENTS

This group of drugs, which includes the salicylates, analine derivatives and pyrazolone derivatives, are known as antipyretics because they have the power to reduce body temperature. According to their

Table 13 The pharmacological properties of antipyretic, antirheumatic and anti-inflammatory drugs

	Analgesia	Antipyretic	Anti-inflammatory	Anti-gout
Salicylates	+	+	+	+
Mefenamic acid	+	+	+	—
Flufenamic acid	—	+	+	—
Paracetamol	+	+	—	—
Phenylbutazone	—	+	+	+

properties they are used to relieve mild to moderate pain, to reduce inflammation in the arthritides and to reduce body temperature in fevers (see Table 13).

Salicylates

Herbal remedies derived from tree bark, leaves and fruit used for the relief of pain, fever and inflammation owe their effectiveness to the salicylates which have analgesic and antipyretic properties. Salicyclic acid, first produced industrially in 1873 has a wide range of uses, though even now its mode of action is not fully understood. The most commonly used member of the group is acetylsalicylic acid (aspirin). This drug, and substances like it, inhibit pain producing substances including bradykinin and other kinins peripherally and by interacting with prostaglandins (see p. 31). Safe and effective, it is widely used by the medical profession and general public alike to relieve minor aches pains and fevers. It is a drug of choice in treatment of chronic arthritis where its anti-inflammatory properties are of considerable importance, but to achieve a satisfactory effect the dose must exceed 3.6 g per day. Lesser doses of 600 mg four to six times daily are required for pain and the main side effect of the drug if given for long periods at high doses is impairment of haemostasis. This is important where patients have a history of peptic ulcer and even in those without such a history a gastric erosion may occur after a small dose of aspirin in susceptible subjects. The irritating effects of aspirin can be avoided or reduced by taking it after food, by using an enteric coated preparation, by combining aspirin with aluminium oxide or by using paracetamol instead for pain relief. The latter drug is commonly prescribed for those with a history of peptic ulcer. Gastric tolerance may also be increased by using benorylate (Benoral), an aspirin-paracetamol ester which breaks down after absorption into aspirin and paracetamol. It may be given as tablets or a suspension twice daily. The fact that paracetamol is released slowly reduces the chance of hepatotoxicity if an overdose is taken.

Apart from its effects on blood clotting mechanisms the toxicity of this group of drugs, salicylism, is characterised by nausea, vomiting and tinnitus, together with respiratory alkalosis produced by hyperventilation due to stimulation of the respiratory centre. In severe poisoning there may also be hypocalcaemia, hypoglycaemia and hypoprothrombinaemia. Allergic responses are uncommon, occurring mostly in those with a history of allergy. The latter reaction includes urticaria, skin rashes, angioneurotic oedema, and on rare occasions a severe form of asthma.

Aspirin is not recommended, other than in single doses, for children under one year of age because of the danger of metabolic acidosis and fatal poisoning which may follow repeated doses.

Despite its effectiveness as an anti-inflammatory anti-pyretic and analgesic drug the toxicity of the high doses of aspirin once used for many patients with rheumatoid arthritis greatly reduced patients' compliance—their willingness to take the drug as prescribed. Nowadays, therefore, aspirin is given to fewer patients with this disease and for most treatment involves the prescription of non-corticosteroidal anti-inflammatory drugs which are better tolerated and taken on fewer occasions each day.

Diflunisal (Dolobid)

This drug has certain chemical similarities to salicylates but is better tolerated. It is long-acting and effective when given twice daily in doses of 250 mg to 500 mg. Diflunisal is used to treat mild to moderate pain, especially pain associated with arthritic or musculoskeletal disorders. It has been compared with aspirin, dextropropoxyphene with paracetamol (Distalgesic) and pentazocine in the treatment of such disorders and is reported to be equally effective. Diflunisal should not be given to patients with an active peptic ulcer or those who have experienced acute asthmatic attacks as a result of aspirin or NSAID ingestion.

Paracetamol

This drug is perhaps the most commonly prescribed analgesic for mild to moderate pain including headache, toothache, rheumatic pain and dysmenorrhoea. Its central role in pain relief owes much to the fact that, unlike aspirin, it does not irritate the gastric mucosa, but, on the other hand it is a less potent anti-inflammatory drug. The analgesic and anti-pyretic properties of paracetamol make it a popular choice for the treatment of colds and influenza. It should not be prescribed for patients with hepatic or renal damage and doses in excess of 10–15 g cause serious, and perhaps fatal, liver damage. The use of the drug in full doses for prolonged periods should be avoided. The usual dose for adults is 0.5 g to 1.0 g up to four times each day.

NON-CORTICOSTEROIDAL ANTI-INFLAMMATORY DRUGS

These drugs, of which there are many, are almost all similar in potency to aspirin but cause fewer and less severe side-effects with the exception of the most powerful members of the group, indomethacin, oxyphenbutazone and phenylbutazone, which should be used only if other less toxic drugs fail to relieve patient's symptoms. The less toxic drugs differ little in potency although there are great variations in the responses of patients to them in terms of side-effects. They are used chiefly to treat minor rheumatic disorders, (mild osteoarthritis and rheumatoid arthritis), and musculo-skeletal disorders; more specifically, sports injuries which often fall into this diagnostic category.

The main side-effects of the non-corticosteroidal anti-inflammatory drugs are gastric irritation, the precipitation of allergic phenomena (rashes, asthma and angioneurotic oedema), headache, vertigo and tinnitus. Therefore caution should be excercised in the case of patients with a history of peptic ulceration, of allergic disorders and those who have hepatic or renal impairment.

Mefenamic acid and flufenamic acid (Ponstan, Meralen)
These anthranilic acid derivatives have been introduced in recent years as antirheumatic agents although their anti-inflammatory properties are minor. Mefenamic acid has analgesic activity similar to that of aspirin though it is less effective. It is given in doses of 250 to 500 mg by mouth three times daily and its toxic effects are similar to those of aspirin though it is less likely to produce intestinal bleeding. Unfortunately it has a tendency to cause diarrhoea which may be severe. Flufenamic acid relieves pain when given in doses of 200 mg three times daily and, like mefenamic acid, it is used to treat milder rheumatic disorders. Its toxicity resembles that of mefenamic acid.

Naproxen (Naprosyn)
A combination of good symptom relief, low incidence of side-effects and administration only twice daily has made this drug one of the most popular for the treatment of rheumatic disorders, musculo-skeletal conditions, and acute gout. The dose range for rheumatic

disorders is 0.5 to 1 g daily in two divided doses, and for acute gout it is 750 mg initially followed by 250 mg every eight hours. It is available as tablets and suppositories (naproxen 500 mg).

Other drugs similar in effectiveness to naproxen but with more gastro-intestinal side-effects are available including, fenoprofen (Fenopron), flurbiprofen (Froben) and ibuprofen (Brufen) which has weaker anti-inflammatory properties but produces fewer side effects. This drug is not suitable for acute inflammatory disorders such as gout and ankylosing spondylitis. Thus, it is clear that the reader has to consider the potency of each drug in terms of its potential for producing analgesia and reducing inflammation weighed against possible side-effects before embarking upon the treatment of any given patient.

Indomethacin (Indocid)

Indomethacin is a drug with anti-inflammatory properties and is used in the treatment of rheumatoid and other chronic arthritic conditions including ankylosing spondylitis. Its potency equals of aspirin. It is also a gastric irritant and may provoke peptic ulceration with haemorrhage or even perforation. Thus it is advisable to begin treatment at a low dose, that is 25 mg twice daily increasing until a therapeutic effect has been gained but not exceeding 150 mg daily. In order to relieve pain at night and the early morning stiffness of sufferers of rheumatoid arthritis and ankylosing spondylitis the drug may be given as a suppository (100 mg), or in a dose of 75 mg to 100 mg orally, or as a retard preparation in a dose of 75 mg. All forms of the drugs should be used at bedtime and it is advisable to take food if using the oral preparations. Suppositories have irritant effects on the rectal mucosa and rectal ulceration with bleeding may occur. Other toxic effects include dizziness and headache and about 10 to 20 per cent of patients taking the drug will experience side effects of some kind.

Phenylbutazone and Oxyphenbutazone (Butazolidin, Tanderil.)

ne which
nflamma-
fly in the
azone and
: irritants
ot exceed
erapeutic
d to situ-
ents have

ERRATUM

page 163: Phenylbutazone and Oxyphenbutazone

Since the proofs of this book went to press the Committee on the Safety of Medicines has decided that the drug phenylbutazone should be restricted to the treatment of ankylosing spondylitis and be limited to use in hospitals only; oxyphenbutazone has been withdrawn totally from use.

failed because they are highly toxic with potentially serious side effects, including gastro-intestinal disturbances such as anorexia, nausea, vomiting, dyspepsia, ulceration, stomatitis and diarrhoea. They may also cause liver and renal damage and precipitate congestive cardiac failure in patients with heart disease or hypertension. Perhaps most serious of all, although uncommon, the drugs may cause agranulocytosis in young patients, or aplastic anaemia in the elderly. With aplastic anaemia in mind regular haematological checks should be made during the treatment of elderly patients.

It should be noted that phenylbutazone is a powerful hepatic microsomal enzyme inducer with a result that its own half-life and that of drugs similarly metabolised, such as barbiturates, are cut by 50 per cent. Moreover as it is bound to plasma protein, phenylbutazone will displace other drugs that are similarly bound and in this way it potentiates the effects of anticoagulants and sulphonamides, at the same time retarding its own excretion.

Azapropazone (Rheumox) and feprazone (Methrazone) are similar in structure to phenylbutazone but less toxic, especially with regard to effects upon the haemopoietic system. They are used in the treatment of the main forms of arthritis, in doses of 300 mg to 600 mg two to four times daily respectively after meals. For the treatment of gout azapropazone is given in a dose of 2.4 g in divided doses over the first 24 hours and then 1.8 g reducing to 1.2 g daily in divided doses.

To conclude, none of the non-corticosteroidal anti-inflammatory drugs gives a lasting cure for rheumatic disorders and their role appears to be one of symptom suppression.

COMMENTS ON THE USE OF ANALGESIC DRUGS

1. Prescribe a drug which is in keeping with the patient's needs. In other words choose a preparation which is of the appropriate potency for the pain experienced and which gives the required level of sedation. Where the circumstances indicate use a drug which has proven value for the relief of particular forms of pain, for example the use of pethidine for relieving renal colic.

2. Anticipate the development of pain or any tendency for it to increase and prescribe an analgesic at times which will ensure the pain is abolished or minimised.

3. Ensure that the patient does not have to ask for analgesics. A regular prescription is preferable to an 'on demand' schedule as it reduces patient's anxiety about availability of drugs.

4. Do not give drugs on a regular basis to patients with chronic pain without checking regularly upon the need for them and their effectiveness.

5. Remember that analgesics have side effects, some of which are sufficiently unpleasant to make patients reject the drugs. Therefore use preparations with the lowest levels of toxicity and prescribe them in doses which give the maximum pain relief with a minimum of side-effects.

6. Remember that pain control does not depend upon the use of analgesics alone. The following groups of drugs are given either to act specifically upon tissues from which pain arises or upon the central nervous system either to depress consciousness or excitability.

a. Antispasmodics, e.g. atropine.
b. Smooth muscle relaxants, e.g. nitrites, alpha and beta blockers.
c. Steroids, e,g, prednisolone and dexamethazone.
d. Anticonvulsants, e.g. carbamazepine and phenylhydantoin.
e. General anaesthetic agents, e.g. nitrous oxide, trichlorethylene, methoxyflurene.

Other agents used in pain relief include tranquillisers, cytoxic drugs, hormones and antibiotics. Pain control may be achieved by other means too which are preferred under certain circumstances, and these include nerve blocks using local anaesthetics, section of sensory nerves, or the destruction of pain nerve fibre pathways in the spinal cord and brain. These and other physical methods of pain relief are discussed in Chapter 17.

15

Psychotropic drugs for pain relief

The relation between pain and emotion has been dealt with in detail elsewhere (Chapter 11) and to summarise there are several situations in which drugs which influence a patient's emotional state through their action on the brain (psychotropic drugs) may be used either alone or in combination with analgesics to reduce or abolish pain. These are:

1. Where there is heightened emotion on the basis of a constitutional predisposition to anxiety which in turn increases the severity of pain arising from an organic source.
2. Where there is intolerable emotion secondary to pain of organic origin.
3. Where pain arises in the absence of a detectable physical cause and where psychological factors are clearly related to its presence.

Psychotropic drugs are classified in the following manner*:

1. Neuroleptics (the major tranquillisers)

a. These drugs are used in the treatment of a wide range of mental disorders: most commonly the psychoses.
b. They produce extra-pyramidal signs such as tremor and rigidity and, as a result, are used in association with drugs which prevent the emergence of these effects (anti-parkinsonian drugs).

Members of the group

a. Phenothiazines, e.g. chlorpromazine.*
b. Thioxanthenes, e.g. thiothixene.
c. Butyrophenones, e.g. haloperidol,* droperidol.*
d. Diphenylbutylpiperidines, e.g. pimozide.
e. Reserpine derivatives, e.g. reserpine.

*Asterisks indicate that a drug is used in pain relief either alone or in combination analgesics.

2. Anxiolytics (the minor tranquillisers)

a. These drugs reduce anxiety, tension and agitation without any appreciable effect on consciousness, though when at first taken, or if taken in high doses, they produce feelings of tiredness and sleepiness. At times they are used to control epileptic fits and some are used as hypnotics, that is, to induce sleep.

b. There is a strong likelihood that the drugs will produce psychological dependence but the development of physical dependence is less common. The drugs produce fewer toxic effects upon the central nervous system than minor tranquillisers.

Members of the group

a. Benzodiazepines, e.g. chlordiazepoxide, nitrazepam, diazepam.*

b. Propanedioles, e.g. meprobamate.*

c. Barbiturates, e.g. sodium amylobarbitone.

3. Antidepressants

a. The antidepressants are used to relieve all forms of depression. The tricyclic antidepressants produce parasympathomimetic effects, such as a dry mouth, constipation, urinary retention, raised intra-ocular pressure and hypotension. The newer antidepressant, mianserin, which is not a tricyclic compound, is devoid of significant peripheral anticholinergic activity and, in fact, produces few unwanted effects apart from drowsiness. The monoamine oxidase inhibitor group produce sympathomimetic effects, chiefly hypertension.

Members of the group

a. Tricyclic compounds, e.g. imipramine,* amitriptyline.*

b. Quaternary compounds, e.g. mianserin.

c. Monoamine oxidase inhibitors, e.g. phenelzine.*

4. Psychostimulants

a. These drugs increase the level of alertness, reduce fatigue and depression.

b. They cause excitement and may precipitate a psychosis and drug dependence.

Members of the group

a. Amphetamines, e.g. dexamphetamine.*

b. Caffeine.

5. Psycholeptics

a. These drugs produce abnormal mental phenomena including changes in perception, hallucinations and delusions.
b. They may precipitate psychotic disorders in predisposed individuals.

Members of the group

a. Lysergic acid diethylamide (LSD)
b. Mescaline
c. Psylocybin
d. Cannabis

MAJOR TRANQUILLISERS

Only two members of the group, the phenothiazines and the butyrophenones have found a regular place in the treatment of pain. Of the former, chlorpromazine (Largactil) is widely used because it produces emotional tranquillity by depression of emotional centres in the brain, by reducing the alerting effect of the reticular formation upon the cerebral cortex thereby lowering its responsiveness, and by potentiating the effect of narcotic analgesic drugs. It also has an anti-emetic effect which is of value where either powerful analgesic drugs or the patient's illness produce vomiting. Although chlorpromazine is of considerable value as an adjunct to analgesics it should be remembered that in very small doses (less than 25 mg) it potentiates pain and also it may produce depression of mood.

When supplementing analgesics, such as dihydrocodeine or pentazocine, a dose of 25 to 50 mg of chlorpromazine is given by mouth or intramuscular injection. A combination of 50 mg of chlorpromazine and 50 mg of pethidine by intramuscular injection produces profound sedation which is of value where minor surgery or painful and unpleasant investigative procedures are to be carried out without the production of unconsciousness as would be the case with a full general anaesthetic.

Other members of the phenothiazine family of drugs, pericyazine (Neulactil) and perphenazine (Fentazin) are used as adjuncts to analgesics and both may act primarily via their powerful anxiolytic properties.

Butyrophenones were mentioned previously in connection with the use of the piperidine derivative of pethidine, fentanyl, for the latter is often combined with droperidol to produce neuroleptanalgesia. In addition to analgesia a profound reduction of emotional activity occurs and this combination of drugs also has anti-emetic properties. It is often used in minor neurosurgical procedures and the doses of the two drugs are droperidol 5 mg and fentanyl 0.1 to 0.2 mg by intravenous injection. This combination of drugs should be given by those with a sound knowledge of them, namely anaesthetists, whereas the combination of chlorpromazine and pethidine is safer to handle and can be used by other doctors.

The major tranquillisers potentiate the sedative effects of alcohol, anaesthetic agents and barbiturates. They can also cause orthostatic hypotension and in large doses they produce extra-pyramidal symptoms which mimic Parkinson's disease. In a few susceptible individuals they may produce such symptoms at very low doses and in the case of long-term use of the phenothiazine anti-Parkinsonian drugs are given in combination with them.

THE MINOR TRANQUILLISERS

The benzodiazepines

Benzodiazepines are the most widely prescribed of all drugs and account for almost 5 per cent of all prescriptions in Britain each year. This group of drugs is widely used to control anxiety and various members of it are given in conjunction with analgesic drugs. In small doses they do not affect cortical function and thus do not impair consciousness in any way, yet by their action upon centres concerned with generation of emotion in the limbic system they produce a sense of calmness and increased tolerance for stress. At higher doses the drugs cause drowsiness. They are metabolised at different rates; some have long half-lives because they are metabolised via several intermediaries (for example, diazepam [Valium], chlordiazepoxide [Librium] and medazepam [Nobrium]). Others are rapidly excreted by the kidneys, have short half-lives and briefer effects, (for example, oxazepam [Serenid-D], lorazepam [Ativan] and temazepam [Normison]). Flurazepam (Dalmane) and nitrazepam (Mogadon), used as hypnotics, have long-lasting effects and their plasma levels rise slowly; in the case of diazepam it may take several weeks to reach a steady plasma level. Differences in their metabolism dictates the use of benzodiazepines. Long-acting compounds, the most popular of which is diazepam, are used to control severe and chronic anxiety. Drugs with a shorter half-life are used to control acute anxiety and feelings of panic (for example, lorazepam and oxazepam). They are also used as adjuncts to relaxation therapy, a technique used increasingly in the management of chronic pain, to provide preoperative medication and to produce deep sedation in minor surgical operative procedures. Benzodiazepines produce psychological dependence and if they are withdrawn suddenly after being taken in high doses over long periods convulsions may occur. Conversely they have anticonvulsant properties and diazepam has a recognised place in the treatment of status epilepticus. The following are the most commonly used members of the group:

1. Diazepam. This drug produces tranquility and euphoria, but it also produces drowsiness which is noticed by a number of patients at an early stage in its use, though this disappears after a few days. As diazepam relieves tension in striated muscle by central action it is of considerable value in the treatment of musculoskeletal disorders. When combined with analgesics, such as paracetamol or a compound tablet of paracetamol and dextropropoxyphene (Distalgesic) the recommended dose is 5 to 10 mg by mouth two to three times daily. Doses of 10 to 20 mg are required only in cases of very severe anxiety and tension. When rapid relief is required the drug should be given intramuscularly in a dose of 5 to 10 mg or by intravenous injection, but when the latter route is being used caution is advised as rapid injection may cause respiratory arrest. This method of administration also produces amnesia for events immediately surrounding the time of injection.

2. Chlordiazepoxide. This was the first member of the benzodiazepines to be produced commercially. It is a good tranquilliser with less tendency to produce drowsiness than diazepam but it does not have the same power to reduce muscle spasm. Like diazepam it too has anticonvulsant properties. The usual dose of the drug is 10 to 20 mg three times daily in states of moderate to severe anxiety.

3. The newer benzodiazepines. These include oxazepam which is a metabolite of diazepam, and lorazepam which is a derivative of oxazepam. These drugs, which have short half-lives, are not noticeably more effective than diazepam but are probably inferior where pain due to muscle spasm is a major symptom. Nevertheless there does seem to be some variation in the sensitivity of individuals to them and should one not be effective it is worth trying other members of the group. Potassium chlorazepate (Tranxene), a long-acting drug, has an advantage over its newer relations because it is given only once daily, preferably just before bedtime in an oral dose of 15 mg. Being a long-acting preparation it provides relief of anxiety for almost 24 hours.

Propanedioles

Use of this group of compounds has been superceded by the development of the benzodiazepines. They tend to produce marked drowsiness and are dangerous if taken in an excessive amount. The most commonly used member of the group, meprobamate (Equanil), acts as both a muscle relaxant and a tranquilliser. In the treatment of pain due to muscle spasm whether secondary to an organic disorder, such as back or limb injury, or where it is the result of psychological activity as in tension headache the recommended dose of meprobamate is 400 mg one to three times daily. Success in treatment is most likely where anxiety and tension are a marked feature of the condition giving rise to muscle spasm, though it is less effective than diazepam. In addition, the drug produces habituation and convulsions may occur on withdrawal after it has been given in high doses for a long period of time.

The barbiturates

These drugs are primarily used as hypnotics or anaesthetic agents, and because of their tendency to produce dependency they have been replaced in the former situation by drugs of the benzodiazepine group. Barbiturate also causes induction of liver microsomal enzymes which hastens its own metabolism and that of other drugs including the common anticoagulants which leads to the reduction of their hypoprothrombinaemic effect. It increases the metabolism of phenytoin, thereby reducing its anticonvulsant effects. There is no reason for using barbiturates in pain relief now that benzodiazepines are available and the fact that it is more difficult for a serious disturbed individual to take his or her life with the latter drugs also increases their value. It should be remembered that barbiturates given for pain relief without analgesics will cause confusion and restlessness.

Antidepressants

Tricyclic antidepressant drugs (the dibenzazepines)

This group of drugs is widely used in the control of depressive illness and they produce relief by action upon the metabolism of brain amines, such as catecholamines and 5-hydroxytryptamine which, as mentioned previously, play a significant part in control of nervous transmission in pathways concerned with pain generation and modulation. In addition they have anticholinergic effects which produce symptoms during treatment, including persistent dryness of the mouth, blurring of vision, constipation and lowering of blood pressure. They affect bladder function by this means too and caution is advised in their use where there is danger of urinary retention in patients with prostatism. As they raise intra-ocular pressure they should not be given to patients with a history of acute glaucoma.

In the treatment of pain tricyclics appear to have an analgesic effect independent of their antidepressant activity. The tertiary amines in this group of drugs are particularly useful in patients who are depressed and have pain as a prominent symptom. In this regard they have been used with success in those who have atypical facial pain, where symptoms of depression are much less prominent than usual being confined to fatigue, mild depression, disordered sleep and weight loss. Where there is a substantial degree of anxiety or agitation as well as depression amitriptyline (Tryptizol) is recommended in an initial dose of 25 mg three times daily, rising to a maximum dose of 50 mg three times daily with 75 mg at night. This drug has both anxiolytic and antidepressant effects. Where fatigue and anergia are prominent imipramine (Tofranil) is used as it has an alerting effect and the recommended dose is 25 mg three times daily, rising to 50 mg three times daily. This drug has been used with success in the treatment of atypical facial pain and in individuals with chronic pain and depression secondary to rheumatoid or osteoarthritis.

The monoamine oxidase inhibitors

This group of drugs produces an increase in the concentration of monoamines such as noradrenaline, dopamine, and 5-hydroxytryptamine in the brain by inhibiting intracellular enzymes of the monoamine oxidase group which effect amine breakdown. In addition to increasing brain amine concentrations monoamine oxidase inhibition also leads to parallel enhancement of the action of these substances peripherally. For this reason any food which contains amines, such as dopa or tyramine may produce serious hypertension if ingested. For example, broad beans contain dopa, and cheese, milk products, yeast products, meat extracts and animal liver contain tyramine. These must be avoided if a monoamine oxidase inhibitor is prescribed. The central effects of narcotic drugs are accentuated and prolonged by monoamine oxidase inhibitors. Drugs used in the treatment of hypertension, for example bethanidine and guanethidine, which cause noradrenaline release from peripheral sympathetic nerve endings if given in high concentrations, for example by intravenous injection, will, in the presence of a monoamine oxidase inhibitor, produce hypertension and excitement. In the presence of a narcotic drug a monoamine oxidase inhibitor may produce excitation, coma, rigidity, hyperpyrexia and fluctuations in blood pressure and it must not be used in combination with them. Where an analgesic has to be given in the presence of monoamine oxidase inhibitor the use of paracetamol is advised. There are also dangers in administering monoamine oxidase inhibitors with a tricyclic antidepressant drug, although in well controlled circumstances this combination is used in the treatment of depression by psychiatrists. The tricyclic antidepressants inhibit uptake of noradrenaline and 5-hydroxytryptamine by central nerve terminals, thereby increasing their concentration and availability to receptor sites; an effect which will be enhanced by a monoamine oxidase inhibitor. Despite all the hazards inherent in the use of monoamine oxidase inhibitors they are often used in the treatment of depressive illness and they appear to be effective in the treatment of 'psychogenic pain' as in the case of phenelzine (Nardil) which is given in a dose of 15 mg three times daily by mouth. In cases where agitation is present chlordiazepoxide (Librium) can be added in a dose of 5 to 10 mg three times daily.

Blockade of serotonin (5-hydroxytryptamine) and pain relief

The evidence for involvement of 5-HT in pain modulation, and knowledge that impaired metabolism of it is part of the biochemical abnormality present in patients with depression and chronic pain, has led to the use of newer antidepressant drugs which are powerful blockers of 5-HT uptake in the treatment of chronic pain. Clomipramine (Anafranil) was the first compound to be developed and has been used successfully in combination with carbamazepine (Tegretol) in the treatment of post-herpetic neuralgia. It has also been used to enhance the effect of analgesics in rheumatic diseases. In both cases doses ranging from 10–25 mg are given at night.

Very recently zimelidine (Zelmid), an even more powerful blocker of 5-HT uptake at pre-synaptic nerve terminals, has become available for general clinical use. It is not a tricyclic antidepressant and its anticholinergic activity is weak. The drug has been marketed as an antidepressant but there are some indications that it will be useful in the treatment of patients with chronic pain.

The psychostimulants

Caffeine is the commonest psychostimulant in general use being taken by virtually every adult in the form of tea, coffee or chocolate. It produces a mild feeling of wellbeing and increases alertness. It is included in very small amounts in certain proprietary mild analgesics and probably has little or no effect upon pain, though it may enhance its severity by increasing cortical arousal.

Amphetamines were widely used at one time to counter depression but their liability to cause dependency and the discovery of more suitable drugs for the treatment of depression has led to a complete ban on their use in the United States, although they are available in Britain for very specific purposes, for example the treatment of narcolepsy. Cocaine, also a drug with a marked tendency to cause dependency, produces mental alertness, indifference to pain, hunger and fatigue. For this reason it is used by South American Indians in Peru and other regions, especially those at high altitudes, where chewing coca leaves enables men to carry heavy loads for long distances in conditions which would otherwise cause considerable fatigue. It is used for pain relief during the terminal stages of malignant diseases sometimes as part of an elixir which contains in addition, diamorphine hydrochloride, ethyl alcohol, sweetened flavouring and chloroform water and which is given regularly at four hourly intervals (see p. 217).

16

Drug dependence and placebos

Dependence on the chemical substances caffeine, nicotine and alcohol, is a feature of everyday life in our society. In addition many people from all walks of life are dependent on minor tranquillisers and sedatives but the use of 'hard' drugs like morphine and heroin is confined to minority groups.

The World Health Organization defined drug dependence in 1969 as follows: 'A state, psychic and sometimes also physical, resulting from the interaction between a living organism and a drug characterised by behavioural and other responses that always include a compulsion to take the drug on a continuous or periodic basis in order to experience its psychic effects and sometimes to avoid the discomforts of its absence. Tolerance may or may not be present. A person may be dependent upon more than one drug'.

The terms tolerance and psychic and physical dependence are further defined:

TOLERANCE

'The phenomenon of dose increase to maintain a drug effect'. This means that a drug when taken repeatedly becomes less effective unless the dose is steadily increased and even then the user reaches a point where further increases in its dose do not produce an improvement in effectiveness.

PSYCHIC DEPENDENCE

'The intense craving and compulsive perpetuation of abuse to repeat the desired effects of a psychotropic drug'. The drugs which have this effect produce feelings of mental wellbeing or euphoria with a reduction of tension which is replaced by a feeling of 'let down' whenever the effects wear off.

PHYSICAL DEPENDENCE

'An adaptive state which manifests itself by intense physical disturbance when the administration of the drug is suspended or when its action is affected by the administration of the specific antagonist'. All drugs which have this effect are depressants of the central nervous system which functions normally only in the presence of the drug once dependency has been established. If they are withdrawn suddenly excitation of the central nervous system occurs which is the opposite effect of the one produced by the action of the drug. Drugs producing physical dependence include morphine and morphine-like substances, some of the tranquillisers, barbiturates and alcohol, however, the ease with which dependency is established varies, being most rapid with the powerful narcotics.

Tolerance and psychic dependence are common to all forms of drug dependence irrespective of the nature of the drug, but physical dependence is not always present, and the degree to which each of these phenomena occurs with different drugs varies.

DEPENDENCE OF THE MORPHINE TYPE

Heroin is used most commonly amongst those dependent on narcotics. It is injected subcutaneously initially and then intravenously (mainlining) as dependency is established. Within weeks of first taking the drug physical dependence occurs and the addict is compelled to inject himself regularly to avoid unpleasant withdrawal effects, which include restlessness, coldness with shivering and pyloerection (cold turkey), watering of the eyes, running of the nose, sweating, abdominal cramps, vomiting and diarrhoea. Sleep is disturbed and cardiovascular collapse may occur. Symptoms reach their peak in two to three days in morphine and heroin dependency, but in only six to twelve hours in pethidine dependency. The effects of the former may persist over two to three weeks and the latter for six to seven days after discontinuation.

The effects of heroin or morphine habituation on the personality are profound, although most of those involved exhibited inadequacies of personality beforehand implying that they had a low level of ability to cope with the problems of everyday life, were liable to seek immediate gratification of their needs and were impulsive. Judgement, self-control and moral standards degenerate under the influence of habituation and much of the person's time becomes centred upon means, often deviant, of obtaining further supplies of the drug. Mortality amongst heroin addicts, who are mostly adolescents and young adults, is high and death occurs either from septicaemia following the use of unsterile equipment for injection, or an overdose of the drug which is often in an impure form when sold illicitly.

Addiction to pethidine is less common than to heroin and those at greatest risk are doctors and nurses because they have direct access to the drug. Cocaine, which is not commonly used clinically nowadays, except by otorhinolaryngologists, is taken as snuff (snow) and in some instances it is mixed with heroin for intravenous injection. Regular use of this drug causes both physical and psychological dependence.

There is great anxiety amongst doctors and nurses that patients will become dependent on narcotics if given to them for treatment of chronic pain. Although this does occur, as has been discovered as a result of investigations in which patients with terminal cancer have been studied, control of habituation in circumstances where life expenctancy is short is possible when the use of narcotics is kept to the minimum in terms of dosage, and when psychotropic drugs and psychological means of support are also available.

THE PLACEBO EFFECT

A placebo (Latin—I will please) has been defined as 'any therapeutic procedure or component of a therapeutic procedure which is given deliberately or which unknowingly has an effect on the patient's symptoms, disease or syndrome, but which is objectively without specific activity for the condition treated'. The placebo effect is defined as 'the changes produced by placebos'.

Placebos are often used in trials of new drugs where the efficacy of an active preparation is compared with an inactive one. Clearly the investigators have to take account of the placebo's effectiveness too and by appropriate designs of drug trials this can be achieved. The action of the placebo depends upon its nature, the situation in which it is given, by whom it is received and the nature of the disorder being treated. In general the placebo effect is most likely to occur in acute disorders where there is a high level of emotional stress and anxiety. Studies of pre-operative anxiety and pain have shown that the more intense these experiences are for the patient the greater will be his or her response to a placebo. For example, Dr Beecher working in the United States reported in 1959 that where severe pain and anxiety coexisted in his patients 40 per cent of them responded favourably to a placebo and 52 per cent to an injection of morphine. But, when levels of pain and anxiety were low the placebo gave relief to only 26 per cent of the patients treated whereas morphine brought relief to 84 per cent. He made the comment that the average level of effectiveness of placebos is about 35 per cent. Younger women and those of lower intelligence, together with those of a stable and extraverted temperament, are most likely to respond to placebos. Contrary to what might be expected individuals with marked neurotic elements in their personality do not respond well. The mode of action of the placebo is related to the doctor-patient relationship and the expectation of the latter from the former together with an unconscious desire on the patient's part to react favourably in the doctor's eyes when treated. Recent experiments indicate that the placebo effect may have a neurophysiological component also and that this consists of the release of endogenous opioid peptides within the central nervous system in response to stimuli which are primarily psychological. It is important that the patient does not realise the nature of the preparation given and in these circumstances the placebo effect may last for some time. Moreover, when told very firmly and with conviction that the treatment will relieve pain success will be much greater than if patients feel that they are part of an experiment designed to determine whether or not a drug or treatment will work. The assurance given with administration of a placebo is accompanied by measurable changes in body functions effected through the autonomic nervous system and neuronal mechanisms; for example alterations in blood pressure and pulse are commonly produced. So powerful is the effect in some cases that drug dependence, even when narcotics are involved, may appear to continue where substitution of an inert intramuscular preparation is tolerated without withdrawal symptoms until the injections are stopped. Thus the benefits gained by patients from a placebo are based upon its effect upon the emotional component of pain and, in addition to the powerful effects of suggestion, it seems possible that psychologically induced changes in levels of opioid peptides play a part in pain relief. Placebos have side effects. The patients may complain of headaches, dizziness and nausea, or symptoms which they developed when taking active preparations earlier for the same disorder. Though uncommon, withdrawal effects have been observed demonstrating the manner in which the psychological dependency upon a treatment may have nothing to do with its pharmacological activity.

The placebo effect is widely used by those in the medical profession, both consciously and even to a greater extent unconsciously, because in the region of 20 per cent of all medicines prescribed regularly are without any known pharmacological action. Nevertheless, there is prejudice against the deliberate use of placebos, which seems inappropriate in view of the inactivity of many of the drugs we use, and it is an attitude which must be dispelled because the primary aim of the doctor is to relieve his patient's symptoms. If he does so he has succeeded in his professional role and his main task should be to understand why, when using any particular treatment whether pharmacologically active or not, it is effective.

17

Local analgesia, nerve blocks and surgical methods of pain relief

Analgesic drugs have their limits when used for the treatment of moderate to severe chronic pain whether it is due to a benign or a malignant lesion. Their possible side-effects, including impairment of consciousness, nausea, vomiting, constipation, respiratory depression and others, may make life thoroughly miserable for the patient where there is either no risk to survival, or where life expectancy can be measured in terms of many months. Moreover, the long-term use of narcotic drugs is to be avoided because of their potential for inducing tolerance and drug dependency. It is very important to remember also that analgesics may not produce complete pain relief even when taken to the limits of their dosage defined by toxicity and the doctor should always be prepared to tell the patients about this possibility. Fortunately alternative methods for pain relief are available for use in certain circumstances being based either on blocking the conduction of nerve impulses which give rise to pain by means of local anaesthetics, or drugs which will destroy nerve fibres (neurolytics), or by cutting the pathways along which impulses pass. These methods should be used earlier rather than later in the course of a chronic painful disorder allowing the more powerful analgesic drugs to be reserved for the final stages of the illness if necessary. They are chiefly used for pain control in malignant diseases face.

Before using any of the techniques to be described the site of pain should be carefully mapped out and the use of a dermatome chart showing the distribution of nerves to various areas of the body is recommended (Fig. 23). Its use aids clear localisation of pain from superficial and deep structures remembering that referred pain from the viscera is felt in the area of skin served by the same segment of the spinal cord which supplies nerves to the organ or tissue concerned.

NERVE BLOCKS USING LOCAL ANAESTHETICS

Local anaesthetic drugs reduce the rate of conduction of impulses by nerve fibres by impeding the flow of ions across the nerve mem-

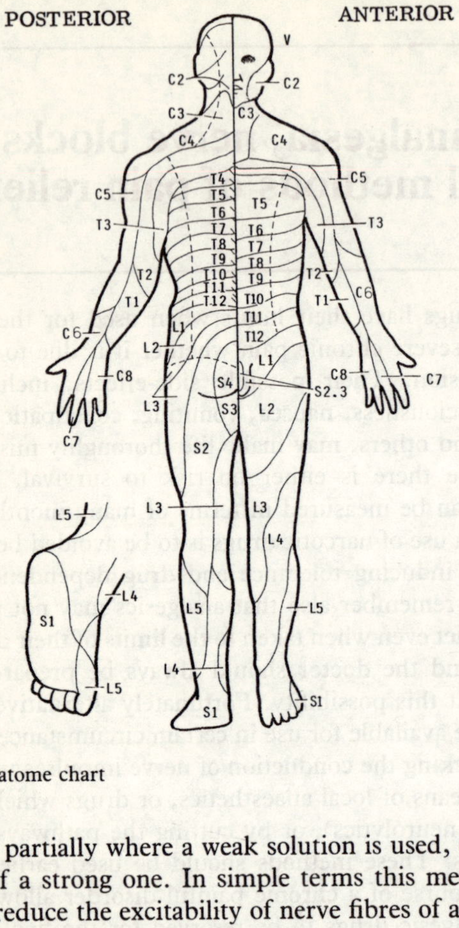

Fig 23. A dermatome chart

brane, either partially where a weak solution is used, or completely in the case of a strong one. In simple terms this means that local anaesthetics reduce the excitability of nerve fibres of all sizes. However, they are most effective where the myelin sheath is thinnest around C fibres, a group chiefly concerned in pain generation. By appropriate adjustment of the concentration of analgesic solutions preferential block of small diameter fibres with sparing of large diameter fibres is achieved. Duration of analgesia depends upon several factors including the molecular structure of the drug, the pH of the solution used, and local tissue factors such as vascularity and the ability of the body to metabolise the drug. In some cases adrenaline, a vasoconstrictor, is added to the solution to slow down absorption from the injection site and to reduce the amount of drug entering the blood stream thereby lowering its systemic toxicity. Combinations of this kind, though still in use, have been replaced to a large extent by new long-acting local anaesthetic drugs.

Local anaesthetics commonly in use at the present time together with some of their characteristics are listed in Table 14.

Table 14 Characteristics of local anaesthetic drugs in common use

Local anaesthetic	Recommended dose mg/kg	Duration of effect	General properties
Lignocaine The most commonly used local anaesthetic for minor surgery	7 (without adrenaline) 3.5 (with adrenaline)	¼ hour (without adrenaline) 1½–2 hours (with adrenaline)	Chemically stable in solution. Rapid onset of action. Good tissue penetration
Bupivicaine Used for prolonged anaesthesia (regional anaesthesia) e.g. post-operative treatment, chest pain in thoracic surgery, treatment of cancer pain	2	5–16 hours	Chemically stable in solution. 4 × power of lignocaine
Amethocaine Used as lozenges to anaesthetise mouth, pharynx and oesophagus. A 0.5 per cent solution is used to anaesthetise the cornea	4	1½–3 hours	Slow onset anaesthesia. Unstable in solution. 10 × power of lignocaine
Prilocaine Used in dentistry, in obstetrics (pudendal blocks), in minor surgery of head, face and neck	10	¼ hour	Similar properties to lignocaine but metabolised more rapidly

THE USE OF LOCAL ANAESTHETICS

Local anaesthetics may be used in the following manner:

1. Topical use

Local anaesthetics are very useful in the relief of itching or pruritis, for anaesthetising the cornea and the mucus membrane of the mouth or urethra and for minor surgical procedures. They are applied as creams, ointments or solutions and they are ineffective where the skin is unbroken. Local anaesthesia for minor surgery, such as the incision of abscesses on the hands, may be obtained by the use of an ethyl chloride spray the rapid evaporation of which produces cooling and insensitivity of the skin for a brief period during which incision is performed. This form of anaesthesia has also been used with a variable degree of success in the treatment of dysmenorrhoea where the spray is applied to the skin of the lower abdomen for a few moments.

2. Local infiltration of nerves

Local anaesthetics may be used in the relief of pain due to minor musculoskeletal disorders where 'trigger spots' are located and an injection is made into them. They are also used in minor surgery, for example in dental procedures, and the duration of anaesthesia in such circumstances is generally more than is required for the operation to be performed. However, it is interesting to note that when injections are given for chronic pain due to trauma the duration of relief is often considerably longer than might be expected, perhaps because freedom from pain allows freer movements of the part of the body concerned and elimination of muscle spasm with removal of pain producing metabolites. As anxiety often plays an important part in maintaining muscle spasm resulting in reduced movement of some part of the body, pain relief may well also ease tension and thereby promote further relaxation and freedom from pain. Occasionally local anaesthetic blocks are used to relieve pain following thoracic surgery in order to avoid the inhibitory effect of the pain upon respiration and thus the development of undersirable pulmonary complications, such as infection.

3. Nerve blocking

In conditions where pain is persistent sensory nerves, or sympathetic ganglia and nerve chains may be blocked with local anaesthetics for short-term relief, or for the identification of nerve pathways involved prior to their destruction with neurolytic agents, or their division by surgical means. Some of the more common uses of nerve blocks are indicated in Table 15.

Nerve blocking is particularly useful where patients are too frail to undergo general anaesthesia and major surgery and the object of the treatment is to block sensory nerves in sufficient numbers to give pain relief yet leaving motor nerves to muscles and viscera functioning. The block may be performed outside or inside the spinal column, the former being preferred where only one or two nerves are to be blocked, and the latter where a wider area of anaesthesia is required (Fig. 24). When a block is performed on sensory nerves outside the spinal column it is usual to use a test injection of local anaesthetic to ensure that the appropriate nerves have been located before injecting a very small volume of the neurolytic agent, which

Table 15 Uses of nerve blocks outside the spinal canal (regional anaesthesia)

Site of block*	Conditions treated
Cranial nerves	
Trigeminal	Trigeminal neuralgia
(Intra and Extra Cranial)	Dental surgery
Cervical nerves	
Phrenic nerve	Intractable hiccough
Cervical plexus	Superficial tumours and cysts of neck
Thoracic nerves	
	Post-operative pain
	Nerve root compression
	Tumour infiltration
Peripheral nerves in limbs	
Elbow, wrist and digital blocks	General and orthopaedic surgery of forearm and hand
Lumbar nerves	
Ilioinguinal nerve	As in thoracic, and nerve entrapment
Iliohypogastric nerve	following hernia repair
Lateral cutaneous nerve of thigh	Meralgia paraesthetica
Sacral and coccygeal nerves	
Pudendal nerves	Obstetric analgesia
Sacro-coccygeal plexus	Coccydynia
Sympathetic nerves	
Stellate ganglion	Causalgia of arm or hand
Coeliac plexus	Pancreatic pain
Sacral plexus	Bladder pain
Dorsal sympathetic chain	Ischaemic necrosis of hands
Lumbar sympathetic chain	Incipient gangrene, Hyperhidrosis
	Ischaemia leg ulcers
	Sympathetic algodystrophies of lower limbs

* In all cases a local anaesthetic block is used as a preliminary procedure to ensure accuracy in placement of a neurolytic agent when a permanent block is required.

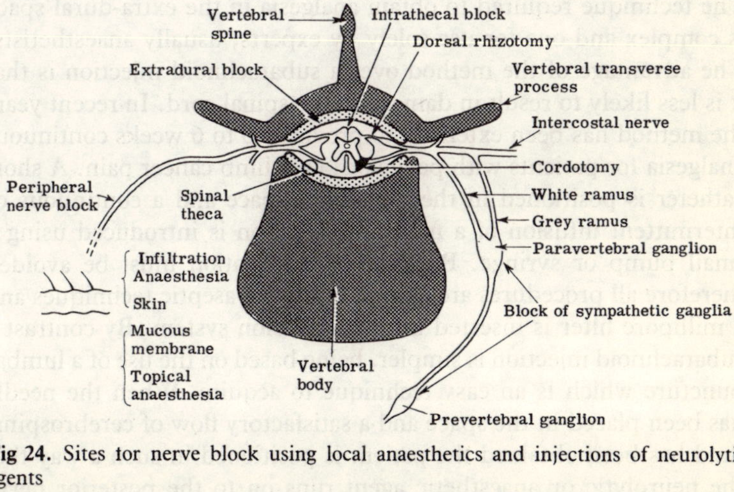

Fig 24. Sites for nerve block using local anaesthetics and injections of neurolytic agents

may be absolute alcohol or phenol. When performing the procedure the injected substance must be placed as close as possible to the nerve using techniques described in more advanced texts.

Occasionally, where patients are obese or anatomical variations lead to misplacement of the needle tip, the operator may fail to produce anaesthesia or obtain only partial relief from pain. Neurolytic blocks are not permanent but often give substantial relief for a period ranging from weeks up to one or two years. In some cases the block is repeated when pain returns, but in others specialised surgical techniques may be employed to give further relief.

Inside the spinal column nerves are blocked either as they pass beyond the layers of the dura mater (an extra-dural block) or in the subarachnoid space (an intrathecal block). The uses of these techniques are summarised in Table 16.

Table 16 Indications for the use of extradural and intrathecal blocks with local anaesthetics

Extradural analgesia	Intrathecal analgesia
Pain of childbirth	Severe pain due to malignant disease
Pain of malignant disease	Pain due to nerve compression following spinal injuries
Pain due to multiple fractures of the ribs	Muscle spasticity in lower limbs
Pain of acute pancreatitis	
Post-operative pain for patients with chronic lung diseases who have had abdominal surgery	

The technique required to obtain analgesia in the extra-dural space is complex and one for use solely by experts, usually anaesthetists. The advantage of the method over a subarachnoid injection is that it is less likely to result in damage to the spinal cord. In recent years the method has been extended to provide up to 6 weeks continuous analgesia for patients with pelvic or lower limb cancer pain. A short catheter is positioned in the extradural space and a continuous or intermittent infusion of a morphine solution is introduced using a small pump or syringe. Bacterial contamination must be avoided therefore all procedures are carried out using aseptic techniques and a millipore filter is inserted into the infusion system. By contrast a subarachnoid injection is simpler, being based on the use of a lumbar puncture which is an easy technique to acquire. When the needle has been placed in the space and a satisfactory flow of cerebrospinal fluid has been obtained the patient is positioned in such a way that the neurolytic or anaesthetic agent runs on to the posterior nerve roots. The former, most often 5 per cent phenol in glycerine, has a higher specific gravity than cerebrospinal fluid so sinks through it to surround the nerve roots to be blocked. Careful positioning of the patient by tilting the table on which he or she is lying is necessary to make sure that the injected fluid does not flow up or down the spinal canal and away from the intended site of action. The maximum effect of phenol occurs within 10 minutes and is usually complete within the hour. As the placement of the neurolytic solution is less precise by this method than any other and because of their powerful effects all nerve fibres may be affected and therefore sensory changes, including numbness and tingling or hyperaesthesia together with some motor weakness or bladder dysfunction, are all possible complications of the procedure depending upon the level at which the injection is made. Fortunately these effects are usually temporary but patients must be warned of the possible side-effects of treatment before embarking upon it. As with any lumbar puncture patients may also experience headache for a few days after treatment, and in some instances there may also be back pain, nuchal rigidity and vomiting (meningism), caused by irritation of the spinal membranes by the chemical agent itself, or infection introduced at the time of injection.

Blocking of sympathetic ganglia or nerve chains by local anaesthetic or neurolytic agents is most commonly used in elderly and debilitated patients with peripheral vascular disease where it helps improve skin blood flow and aids recovery from ischaemic necrosis. Ischaemic muscle pain may also be abolished in some cases too but surgical methods are preferable for relief in cases of this kind. The technique is also used occasionally to relieve causalgia and the severe pain caused by upper abdominal cancer, especially of the pancreas.

Inhalation analgesia

Nitrous oxide is a good analgesic agent and a mixture containing 25 per cent of the gas with 75 per cent oxygen gives a level of post-operative pain relief comparable with that of morphine and very little disturbance of consciousness. A commercial mixture of 50 per cent nitrous oxide and 50 per cent oxygen (Entonox) is available in easily portable cylinders and used by patients to relieve peaks of severe pain that can be anticipated; for example, during the dressing of burns, changing of post-operative dressings, the removal of thoracotomy drains and during physiotherapy for the chest following thoracic surgery. Entonox is used by midwives to control pain late in the second stage of labour when contractions of the uterus are frequent. Trichlorethylene (Trilene) is also used as an inhalation

Table 17 Neurosurgical techniques used to control pain

Level in the nervous system	Operative procedure	Indications for use
Peripheral nerve	Neurectomy	Neuralgias, e.g. meralgia paraesthetica
Dorsal nerve roots	Rhizotomy	Chronic pain in thoracic and abdominal walls
Spinal cord	Open cordotomy Percutaneous Cordotomy	Chronic pain, especially of malignant disease, in arms, trunk and legs
	Electrical stimulation of posterior columns	As above
Brain	Brain steam Tractotomy	As above and where pain is in neck or face
	Electrical stimulation of central grey matter of brain stem, and lateral hypothalamus	As above and also where pain originates from damage to thalamus
	Thalamotomy	
	Leucotomy	Chronic pain with gross agitation uncontrolled by other means

analgesic for this purpose, though less often than Entonox, to cover pain in the other situations mentioned. The mixture used for analgesia contains 0.5 per cent trichlorethylene w/v in air.

SURGICAL RELIEF OF INTRACTABLE PAIN

The surgeon's role in pain control depends upon techniques that have been devised to divide the pathways along which impulses giving rise to pain pass. The levels of the nervous system where this may be carried out are listed in Table 17 and of the techniques listed the one most commonly used is cordotomy.

Dorsal rhizotomy (division of dorsal nervel roots)
Surgeons do not cut peripheral mixed nerves to relieve pain as this would cause extensive sensory loss and motor weakness. However, the dorsal nerve roots which carry sensory fibres only are sometimes cut if the area in which pain occurs can be related easily to a small number of nerve roots. Generally surgery is confined to nerves supplying the thorax or abdomen; sensory loss is not important in these regions, whereas sensory denervation of the limbs or of the face will in the former case produce a useless limb and in the latter a sensation of numbness which may be objectionable to the patient. The conditions treated by dorsal rhizotomy include nerve compression pro-

duced by mechanical distortion or disease of the spinal column, or where there is pain after chest surgery, and occasionally in post-herpetic neuralgia though this does not respond well to this form of treatment. In order to obtain complete pain relief in one dermatome the nerve roots to three of four adjacent ones must be cut in view of the extensive overlap that exists between the territories of sensory nerves.

Antero-lateral cordotomy

The anterior columns of the spinal cord carry many of the afferent fibres concerned in the conduction of nerve impulses giving rise to pain (see Chapter 1). In a cordotomy the surgeon divides one or other and occasionally both the anterior columns in the most lateral parts where the lateral spinothalamic tracts are located. The destruction may be carried out at operation under direct vision, (an open cordotomy), or by means of a needle which is inserted into the tracts with the destruction of tissue by the generation of heat or the use of a freezing device, (percutaneous cordotomy). The former requires a general anaesthetic and major surgery to expose the spinal cord. As most patients in severe pain for whom this type of procedure is carried out are very ill and debilitated percutaneous cordotomy is preferred as it is performed under local anaesthetic only, and in addition the patient is sufficiently conscious to be able to give the surgeon information about the effects of stimulation in the cord during the procedure. This enables him to place his destructive lesion with great accuracy producing pain relief without any other appreciable abnormality. After cordotomy, which is usually performed in the upper cervical region in the case of percutaneous cordotomy, or in the cervical or upper thoracic region if an open cordotomy, the patient loses sensation of pain, heat and cold on the opposite side of the body. The level of analgesia for a cordotomy carried out at the 1st or 2nd cervical segment usually begins about the 3rd or 4th thoracic dermatome. If treatment is satisfactory, which is the case in about 80 per cent of patients, pain relief is complete and instantaneous. The duration of relief varies and may last one or two years. Therefore as cordotomy is often carried out in the last months of life many patients are pain-free until they die. Bilateral cordotomy is occasionally performed but is avoided if possible as it may produce a state in which the patient is unable to breathe unless he or she makes a conscious effort the (Ondine syndrome). A bilateral cordotomy may also produce bladder dysfunction. Therefore, the indications for cordotomy are the presence of severe unilateral pain in the lower or upper limbs, thorax, abdomen or pelvis. Bilateral pain is seldom treated this way for the reasons mentioned. However, relief of unilateral pain occasionally unmasks pain on the previously symptom-free side of the body in which case the surgeon may choose to carry out a second cordotomy at a later date. Because the descending corticospinal tracts are also in the antero-lateral quadrant of the spinal cord motor weakness may be produced on the side of the cordotomy. Fortunately however this is usually transient, especially where percutaneous cordotomy is carried out and the operator is able to ensure that he is not damaging the motor tracts before making a destruction lesion.

The immediate effectiveness of percutaneous stereotactic cordotomy is evident from the results of various reported series which reveal that the unilateral procedure gives complete pain relief to 90–95 per cent of patients. This figure falls gradually but a final figure of approximately 85 per cent can be expected in the hands of skilled neurosurgeons and anaesthetists. About 10 per cent of patients experience motor weakness after operation but only 2 per cent do not recover. Other post-operative problems occur occasionally including dysaesthesia (marked in 1 per cent of patients) and urinary retention (only after bilateral cordotomy).

Cordotomy is not carried out where phantom limb pain is present because loss of sensation in a limb stump prevents the patient from wearing a prosthesis as he or she would be quite unaware of the damage that could be caused by it.

Brain stem tractotomy, operations on the thalamus and leucotomy

Using the technique of stereotactic surgery which enables them to locate any given area within the brain with precision, neurosurgeons are able to destroy nerve tracts along which stimuli giving rise to pain pass, to make lesions in the sensory relay stations for pain fibres in the thalamus, (the postero-lateral and centro-median nuclei), and to destroy the fronto-thalamic connections bilaterally (leucotomy), which diminishes the emotional component of pain without destroying its sensory element. They may also achieve similar results by making destructive lesions in other parts of the limbic system, for example in the cingulum. All the forms of treatment mentioned require a very high degree of surgical skill, are time consuming and carry the risk of physical and mental complications. For example, in the case of operations upon the postero-lateral nuclei of the thalamus the patient may be left with altered sensation either in the form of increased or decreased sensitivity to noxious stimuli and sometimes with worse pan than before operation. In the case of operations on the centro-median nuclei of the thalamus pain relief without sensory changes is more readily achieved. Apart from these factors the operations are disappointing in terms of their success in bringing pain relief. At present they seem often to be performed as a last resort and the judicious use of drugs, nerve blocks or cordotomy are the most frequent forms of treatment given to relieve patients with chronic pain.

CUTANEOUS ELECTRICAL STIMULATION AND ELECTRICAL STIMULATION OF THE POSTERIOR COLUMNS OF THE SPINAL CORD

Within the past few years attempts have been made to modulate pain using techniques based upon the 'gate theory' put forward by Melzack and Wall in 1965, (see page 23). We are all aware that pain, especially acute pain, may be relieved partially or totally by firmly rubbing the damaged area of the body for several minutes and neurologists and others dealing with amputees have noticed a rather similar phenomenon, namely that the application of a vibrator to a limb stump will relieve or abolish phantom limb pain in some cases. Thus, the everyday findings of laymen and clinicians indicate that a substantial increase in the input of sensory activity to the central nervous system from a damaged area of the body in certain circumstances reduces pain. Electrical stimulation of the skin has a similar effect brought about by the low intensity, high frequency output of a stimulator upon Aβ mechanoreceptors, (Fig. 14). Table 18 shows the value of transcutaneous neural stimulation (TNS) in the treat-

Table 18 Variations in the level of response of different painful disorders to treatment by transcutaneous neural stimulation (TNS)

Good response	Low to moderate level of response	No response
Causalgia	Peripheral neuropathy	Pain without an obvious physical basis but a clear psychological component
Amputation stump pain	Chronic, diffuse cervical and back pain	Chronic diffuse abdominal pain
Sciatica	Post herpetic neuralgia	Pain associated with paraplegia, pain due to arachnoiditis, cancer and post-radiation pain. Thalamic pain
Arthritis (e.g. osteoarthritis of knee)	Trigeminal neuralgia	

ment of pain and reveals that it is most successful when used for the relief of pain arising from damage to peripheral nerves.

The stimulating electrodes are placed over the painful area and the current is passed for two to ten minutes. If effective the pain is replaced by a sensation of warmth or tingling in most patients and for several minutes after the current has been switched off the previously painful area may be partially or totally numbed. The duration of pain relief varies. In some cases it lasts as long as six to eight hours and yet in others relief is only obtained when the stimulator is in constant use. As the devices are very small they are easily carried in the pocket, or on a belt, and the electrodes can be kept in position for many hours without ill effects. The benefits of this treatment, if successful, are considerable. Patients no longer require any form of analgesic drugs, the mobility and function of the previously painful part is increased and a sense of wellbeing and confidence is restored, no doubt helped by the fact that patients also find that for the first time in months or years they are able to sleep comfortably.

Transcutaneous electrical stimulation should not be administered to patients with cardiac pacemakers or during pregnancy. Electrical stimulation of the dorsal columns of the spinal cord through which large diameter fibres said to be involved in the process of modulating pain pass, will also abolish pain. However, electrodes must be implanted in the dura mater or directly over the cord itself, a process which entails a major operation and its attendant risks. Recent advances in design have led to the production of flexible electrodes which are introduced into the extradural space via a large gauge needle after the manner of performing a lumbar puncture, with the addition of radiological techniques to ensure that the stimulator lies at the correct level. This form of stimulator is used for very short periods only, chiefly as a means of assessing the potential value of a long-term implant. The electrodes are activated by a stimulator which is either attached to them or which is operated by remote control. In either event the cost and possibility of complications is far higher than with cutaneous stimulation. Therefore, at the present time the latter form of treatment is preferred. Indeed when the advantages and disadvantages of the two techniques are compared the much simpler and safer cutaneous stimulation technique seems to be superior.

HYPOPHYSECTOMY

For reasons that are not well understood abolition of the pituitary gland's functions brings almost immediate pain relief in women with bone metastases from primary carcinoma of the breast, and men with metastatic carcinoma of the prostate. Similar results are obtained with adrenalectomy and removal of the gonads or the use of androgens in females and oestrogens in males. The pituitary gland is destroyed by one of four methods, of which the first is most commonly used:

1. By the introduction of a cryogenic probe, through the nasal cavities and sphenoid sinuses into the pituitary fossa. The gland is destroyed by freezing it with liquid nitrogen circulated through the tip of the probe.
2. By the implantation of radioactive substances, e.g. yttrium, in the gland using the method of approach described in 1.
3. The destruction of the gland under the surgeon's direct vision after performing a craniotomy.
4. Chemical hypophysectomy—destruction of the pituitary gland by an injection of absolute alcohol using the method of approach described in 1.

18

Psychological techniques used in pain relief

The use of drugs and surgical methods for relieving pain has been discussed at length and it will have become clear that appreciation of the psychological principles of the doctor-patient relationship is important if the potential for relief is to be fully exploited. Most doctors are aware of this but few consciously work upon the emotional aspects of their relationship with the patient with the aim of providing a balanced form of management, taking account of biological, psychological and social factors. In this section the treatments described—psychotherapy, hypnosis, acupuncture and manipulation of the social milieus—are sometimes used alone and often in association with physical methods.

PSYCHOTHERAPY

Psychotherapy is defined as any form of treatment which is based chiefly upon verbal communications with the patient in contrast to the use of drugs or physical treatment. The therapy may involve only the patient and the therapist (individual psychotherapy), or be conducted with groups of patients who have similar emotional disorders (group psychotherapy). If therapy is based upon treatment at frequent intervals, for example daily for four days or more each week, as in psychoanalysis, it is said to be intensive. However, it is more usual for patients to attend less often, for example weekly for six months to a year, and to undergo brief psychotherapy. The different forms of psychotherapy and their use in the treatment of pain are as follows:

Supportive therapy

The basis of this form of treatment is that the therapist listens carefully to the patient's conversation showing understanding and expressing concern if appropriate, as the latter is encouraged to put forward problems, conflicts and anxieties. Reassurance and advice are given and the therapist may use his own experiences in life to help the patient gain a clearer understanding of his situation. This form of therapy is frequently used consciously or otherwise by many doctors and is of considerable value in dealing with patients who have organic disorders and, in particular, in acute painful illnesses.

Although special techniques are seldom required when treating acute pain, the thoughtful doctor uses his understanding of the patient's illness and its effects to gain maximum benefit from treatment. Acute illnesses produce anxiety and a sense of disorganisation for the patient who actively seeks his or her doctor's support in so far as the latter is able to restore a sense of orderliness by labelling the disorder, describing its course and treatment, carrying out the treatment and giving an indication about the eventual outcome. This provides both a new self-image for the patient and brings the promise of relief which, in turn, leads to the collaboration of the patient with the doctor and the establishment of a 'treatment contract' between them the basis of which is that the doctor will get the patient back to good health. It should be remembered that patients who are acutely ill need to regress, that is to turn from adult to more primitive childish behaviour, and should be allowed to do so as a protective step whilst in a situation where they are unable to cope alone with the implications of their illness or injury. Such behaviour, though normal, should not be prolonged. By contrast there are some patients who fail to use this protective mechanism and continue to carry more responsibility than is desirable or good for them once they have become ill.

Following the principles of supportive therapy at an early stage the doctor should give the patient a simple factual explanation of the illness, the treatment he intends to carry out, and his expectations about the outcome, being honest about any unpleasant effects that the treatment may bring, for example the fact that pain occurs after surgery but that it will be minimised if not abolished by the use of pain-killing drugs. From time to time acute disorders lead to permanent changes in the way the body functions or to some form of persistent disability as, for example, after bowel surgery where a colostomy is established, or following the amputation of a limb. In these circumstances the doctor must anticipate the likelihood of problems and prepare the patient for them, therefore a patient must never awaken from surgery to find that a major physical reconstruction or amputation, has taken place without prior discussion of the possibility. Patients' relatives also suffer disruption of their lives and experience anxieties about the patients' welfare, the future of the family and the problems ahead if long-term medical care or supervision is required. Therefore, they too should be involved in discussions about treatment and its outcome with the doctor remembering that difficulties surrounding acute or chronic painful disorders will only emerge if he listens giving the patient or relatives time to express their own feelings and most important of all, attempts to understand them. It is important to remember that sufferers of chronic pain and their relatives both become sensitive to any actions on the part of doctors, nurses or others involved in treatment that, rightly or wrongly, appear to signal rejection.

Suggestive therapy

This form of therapy is based on the use of direct suggestion in an attempt to help resolve patients' difficulties and conflicts. The most intensive kind of treatment used is hypnotherapy, described on page 199.

Interpretative therapy

This form of therapy is more complex in its structure, more time consuming and chiefly carried out by psychiatrists or psychologists who have undergone special training in the techniques involved. It is directed towards helping the patient understand the meaning of his or her symptoms. It involves the interpretation of their difficulties in everyday life and often a detailed analysis of the patient's emotional relationship to the therapist because they tend to displace on to the latter feelings and ideas which originated in relationships with others. Through analysis of the therapist-patient relationship and the changes that occur in it with time the significance of various aspects of earlier emotional events to psychologically determined physical symptoms, such as pain, may be examined.

This form of therapy is chiefly used in chronic painful disorders and the patients selected for treatment have the following general characteristics:

1. Their emotional response to physical illness is abnormal in its intensity or duration.
2. They have a pain for which an organic cause cannot be found, or which from the outset is recognised as being psychologically determined.
3. They are intelligent and have sufficient awareness of their own 'inner mental life' to allow the development of a working relationship with a psychotherapist.

In Britain and the United States most clinicians practising interpretative psychotherapy use techniques based upon the psychoanalytic concepts formulated by Sigmund Freud. As the treatment is specialised and not normally carried out by the surgeon or physician, but by a specialist in psychotherapy, the process of referral often precipitates initial difficulties for the therapist of which doctors should be aware. For example, some patients become angry at having to see a psychotherapist because they or their friends and relatives regard the move as a rejection by the physician or surgeon, or a move which carries the implication that their pain is imaginary, or that they are incurable. Some even feel that they are regarded as 'mental' or 'mad'. Thus the patients arrive for their first consultation with considerable feelings of hostility mingled with bewilderment and, in many cases, a fear that referral means discontinuation of analgesics and other drugs or treatments which have formed an essential part of their maintenance of the 'sick role'. Some patients refuse to attend for treatment and in such cases the physician, surgeon, or family doctor, should not abandon them but give continued support and time for the individual to come to terms with the idea that psychological therapy may be helpful. It must be remembered that at this stage of his or her painful illness the patient has experienced several failed treatments, feels he or she has been rejected by the doctors and, usually, feels miserable, demoralised and helpless. Often there is a sense of lost self-confidence and anger and, therefore, it is no surprise that referral to a psychiatrist seems like the final act of rejection on the part of the family doctor or hospital specialist who has failed to relieve suffering usually regarded as entirely physical in origin by the patient.

If the first appointment is kept and initial hostility dealt with satisfactorily, the therapist is then often faced with a patient who concentrates almost exclusively upon repeated descriptions of his or her pain and the history of its development. At the same time he or she makes constant open or thinly disguised appeals for continued physical treatment of some kind which are regarded as the only acceptable way to recovery. This phenomenon, known as 'resistance', indicates that the patient is not able to discuss deeper feelings at this point. In such circumstances the therapist often has to accept the patient's need for analgesics and other drugs, making sure, however, that the doses are kept to the normal level prescribed.

Where therapy progesses satisfactorily beyond this point, and this usually means that the therapist has dealt with the patient's anxieties about releasing feelings and has established a good relationship, the latter begins to talk more freely about emotional problems and less about pain and physical treatments, often discontinuing them spontaneously. He or she begins to appreciate the relationship between pain and emotion and, in particular, to realise that pain is a symbol of mental suffering, that it is what might be called, 'mental pain', and that it is not an indication of a physical disease, nor that it is imaginary. They may also begin to realise that they use their pain to manipulate relationships with others. In other words they are made aware of the contribution of physical, mental and social factors to their behavior. During therapy the relationship between the patient and the therapist deepens with a gradual decrease in the patient's tensions, strengthening of his or her problem-solving ability, an increase in self-esteem, and a positive attitude towards productive goals in relationships with others. Quite often the therapy stops at this point with the therapist making sure that the patient understands that a return of pain or an increase in its severity should be seen first as a possible resurgence of old difficulties, or the appearance of new ones which, if dealt with satisfactorily, will lead to the reduction of symptoms once again. It is common for patients to continue to have pain which fluctuates in this way and a doctor who refers a patient for psychotherapy should not expect either complete relief, nor permanent relief for his patient and this applies both to situations where there has been disease or injury, or where evidence of physical abnormalities cannot be found. The reader should also bear in mind that often a close relative is involved in a complex emotional relationship with the patient and that this plays an important part in the patient's response to therapy. In some cases the relative will undermine, consciously or otherwise, the therapist's attempts to relieve pain. In fact, certain relationships are 'cemented' in a bizarre fashion being maintained only by continual suffering on the part of one of its members. Therefore, occasionally, the therapist may decide to 'permit' his patient to keep symptoms but hopefully at a level that allows more domestic and social activity and less dependence on medicines. One of the most common problems of this type is based upon marital difficulties. For example, a woman's chronic pain may represent a response to her inability to gratify her needs for dependence in other ways, to her ambivalence towards her own or her husband's sexual needs, or to suppressed anger and frustration with a husband who has had an extramarital relationship. The presence of highly dependent, hypochondriacal or hysterical personality traits act as a fertile setting for the 'somatisation' of emotional problems and in particular the development of chronic pain that does not have an obvious or significant physical basis.

At times the patient fails to relinquish his or her intense interest in the somatic complaints that present initially. This may be due to persistent high levels of tension arising out of the ease with which the patient becomes frustrated and angry when emotional needs, which are considerable, are not met by the therapist who is seen as a powerful and authoritarian figure. Although such hostile feelings may be unconscious, or suppressed, they are important in the relationship with the therapist and other doctors who have attempted treatment of a physical kind because, especially in the case of the latter, they often provoke the doctor to retaliate in some way because of his inability to control pain. For example the doctor, may develop feelings of anger and frustration and feel that his professional role is being challenged with the result that he may punish his patient by threats that treatment will be withheld or discontinued, and by retreating into the use of purely physical means of treatment.

Group psychotherapy

This form of treatment is usually carried out by a psychologist or psychiatrist on patients who are attending a Pain Clinic, or who are inpatients. The method is used for reasons of economy where large numbers of patients require treatment, or where it is felt that a patient will have difficulties in establishing a relationship with a therapist, or where the therapist prefers to let his patient examine and improve his ability to relate normally to others in the presence of those who have similar problems to his own. Other advantages to be gained from this form of therapy, which is very popular with those treating patients with pain problems or psychosomatic disorders in the United States especially, are that the patient's sense of being alone, of being alienated and of being different are reduced in the presence of others with similar physical, emotional and social difficulties. Dependence on the therapist is reduced and patients are often more willing to accept interpretation of their difficulties and advice about management of them from their peers than from a single therapist. Their fears of serious disease, lifelong incapacity to cope with stresses, drug dependence and other problems can be freely ventilated and the group gives support or criticises quite readily when appropriate. This may well add considerable support to the doctor's own efforts in treatment carried on outside the group, with the latter helping the patient to establish healthy goals to which he or she gradually works, thereby obtaining greater satisfaction from work, leisure and personal relationships. They are prevented from developing unrealistic hopes about recovery and what they will eventually be able to achieve, also their preoccupation with themselves is reduced as part of developing contact with others.

MODIFICATION OF BEHAVIOUR BY OPERANT CONDITIONING

This approach to the treatment of chronic pain is based on a view that all forms of behaviour, including that associated with pain, are learned, and that faults in the learning process may be modified or corrected without necessarily involving direct intervention with a patient's deeper mental life. In other words, if the patient in pain is behaving in a way that is currently or ultimately to his or her disadvantage in terms of coping effectively with work and interpersonal relationships this should be amenable to correction by system of rewards for 'good behaviour' and punishments for 'bad behaviour'. As in the case of group psychotherapy this form of treatment is most effective if used in pain centres where patients attend frequently or are resident, and in some cases both modification of behaviour using this method and group psychotherapy are carried out simultaneously.

Fordyce has described the principles of the technique in detail and they are as follows:

1. Behaviour is governed by its consequences. Those consequences which increase the occurrence of a particular form of behaviour are known as positive reinforcers, and those which decrease it as negative reinforcers.

2. Behaviour associated with pain can be maintained, enhanced or extinguished by appropriate use of reinforcers. Positive reinforcers include attention, sympathy, concern, rest and analgesic drugs. Undesirable aspects of behaviour, for example lying in bed instead of performing some domestic task, the making of frequent requests for analgesics or complaining about pain, are dealt with by the withdrawal of positive reinforcers, returning them only when the patient follows a desirable pattern of behaviour which has been worked out with him or her beforehand as part of the therapy programme. In practice this means that desirable forms of behaviour will be noticed, complimented and encouraged, whereas undesirable behaviour will be ignored. This approach has been used with some success in the United States to help chronic invalids in pain to achieve higher levels of self-esteem, reduced levels of pain and reduced requirements for analgesic drugs. It has also helped them develop realistic and satisfying physical, emotional and social goals. Another situation allied to the treatment of pain is that of drug dependency and this has also been tackled both by the use of operant conditioning and group psychotherapy, either separately or together.

HYPNOTHERAPY

Hypnosis is a state of mind in which the subject shows increased susceptibility to suggestions made by the hypnotist, whether in a therapeutic setting or in other circumstances. It seems that a hypnotic trance is most easily induced in subjects who have a highly developed ability to produce the mental images suggested to them by the therapist and that hypnotisability is an aspect of each person's make-up that does not change appreciably from childhood to old age. The hypnotist can vary the response of the subject by inducing a state which varies from a mild degree of hyper-suggestibility to one in which physical changes, such as anaesthesia or paralysis, can be induced. In laboratory work it seems that the individuals who have not previously experienced hypnosis do, when hypnotised, report a marked reduction in pain on the application of noxious stimuli and it seems that the amount by which the pain is reduced is positively correlated with their degree of hypnotic susceptibility. Interestingly, although subjects report less pain or no pain at all on the application of noxious stimuli the usual physiological responses to pain, including changes in heart rate and respiration, can be observed. Thus, it is felt that hypnosis is a process by which brain mechanisms are manipulated and though the way in which this happens is not understood it seems to involve preventing sensory activity, which has excited activity in autonomic centres on its way towards the cortex, from reaching consciousness.

Hypnotically induced analgesia has been used for many years in dentistry, childbirth, the relief of pain from burns and various surgical operations. There is no doubt that a number of patients when hypnotised can endure physical experiences which would normally be painful, but stringent investigations of the use of hypnosis reveal that it is probably less effective than might be hoped, especially when used to relieve pain in surgical procedures. Those who have investigated this matter agree that the use of pharmacologically induced analgesia is more reliable and consistent. One extensive review of hypnotherapy concluded that pain at operation is rarely completely abolished and that patients tend to minimise what they experience because they wish to fulfil the hypnotist's expectation of them. Thus, hypnosis has its limitations and in practice approximately only 20 per cent of patients are highly susceptible to the technique, though this number can be increased a little by training and practise. However, these comments are not intended to indicate that mild or moderate pain cannot be abolished or reduced by hypnosis, as the state of calm, of relaxation, and of distraction from noxious stimuli, is of benefit where there is marked intensification of fear of pain by unpleasant memories of similar past events.

The main indication for hypnosis in the treatment of chronic disorders seems to be where pain is not severe and where anxiety and tension play a significant part in provoking or maintaining the symptom. Although only 20 per cent of the population are easily hypnotised many more benefit from the state of relaxation induced by the therapist. Moreover, all skilled hypnotherapists consciously employ psychotherapeutic techniques in their management of patients with chronic pain. The effects of therapy may be extended by teaching the patient the art of self-relaxation and, if possible, autohypnosis—processes which can be carried out as often as necessary and which give patients the important feeling of being able to exert some control over their own body and symptoms.

BIOFEEDBACK

The process of biofeedback consists of providing patients with information about changes in physiological functions of which they are normally unaware. The 'target' system or structure having been selected (for example, the vascular system or a muscle body) its activity is monitored electronically and 'fed back' to the patient as an easily recognised signal. For example, changes in blood pressure or in muscle tone may be registered as a variable tone, or a series of clicks heard through headphones, or as a signal on a visual display unit (VDU) watched by the patient. Strange though it may seem patients can be taught to alter various physiological functions by concentrating upon the 'feedback' and altering it by mental effort alone. For example, using electromyographic recordings from the frontalis muscles, headaches due to muscle tension are relieved if the patient is able to relax the muscles by concentrating upon reducing the signal frequency relayed from them to a VDU. Biofeedback has also been used to treat patients with low back pain, dysmenorrhoea, cervical pain, the pain of peptic ulceration and post-traumatic headache. However, critics of the technique have pointed out that the attentions of the therapist and relaxation cannot be divorced from the effects of mental attempts to alter the feedback signals and therefore from the success of treatment. In fact, there is ample evidence to show that relaxation is as effective as biofeedback in the treatment of painful disorders—it is also cheaper too!

ACUPUNCTURE

Acupuncture is very popular nowadays amongst doctors who specialise in relieving pain and its appearance in Western medicine probably reflects a mixture of curiosity and a need to continue exploring methods of pain relief. The development of the 'gate theory' of pain has almost certainly played a part too as many see the effects of a pain modulating system of this type as the basis of the analgesia produced by acupuncture; especially since the recent discovery that acupuncture increases levels of opioid peptides in the central nervous system.

Acupuncture was first developed in China. Faith in its effectiveness amongst the ancient Chinese was closely interwoven in their view of the origin and early history of the universe and in the maintenance of its equilibrium. The technique was developed on the basis of Chinese theories of anatomy, physiology and philosophy and was described in the 'Nei-ching-Su Wen', a medical text of 3000 years ago and one of the oldest in existence. It involved piercing one or more 'acupoints' on the body, of which there were 365, and through them one or more of twelve channels or meridians. The acupoints represented specific diseased organs and piercing them allegedly permitted the release of evil air which had caused stagnation of the blood. Performance of the procedure was strickly governed by reference to the weather and setting of the moon, and the atmosphere surrounding it was heightened by ceremony and ritual.

The purpose of traditional acupuncture was maintenance of equilibrium in the individual reflecting the Chinese cosmogeny of the time. This was achieved by balancing two states of the body, the yin or female, passive state, and the yang or active, male state. Acupuncture is widely practised in China today and its use together with other elements of traditional Chinese medicine was recommended by the late Mao Tse-tung. It has been combined with Western medical practises and the result is an interesting marriage of diagnostic and therapeutic concepts and techniques. For example if, in the terms of traditional Chinese medicine, the patient is in the yang state he may be prone to headache, anxiety and hypertension. Whereas if he is in the yin state to obesity, lethargy and depression. Acupuncture for pain relief is performed using fine stainless steel needles, two forms of which are shown in Figure 25. Longer needles are used in well covered areas of the body and shorter ones over bone. The needle is inserted into the appropriate acupoint by reference to a meridian map then twirled between finger and thumb, or stroked to produce vibration, or stimulated by a small electric

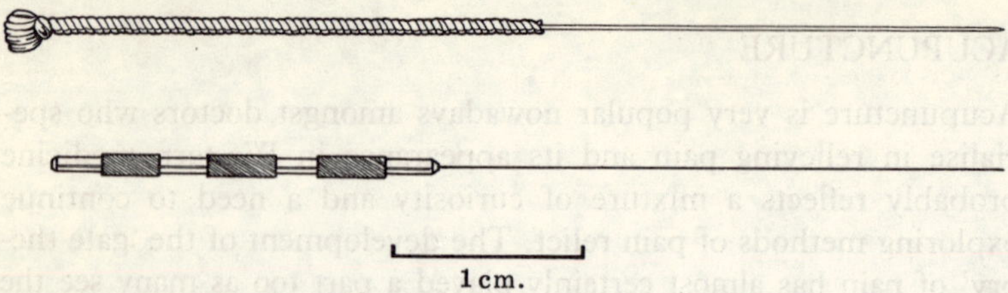

Fig 25. Types of acupuncture needles

current, until the pain disappears. This period varies from a few seconds to 15 to 20 minutes according to the chronicity of the pain and its intensity.

The mode of action of acupuncture has excited much speculation and some experimentation. There are several factors to be considered when attempting to explain its effect, which is considerable, for in China it is reported that 90 per cent of patients are kept free from pain during minor and major surgical operations where it is frequently used in place of general anaesthesia. Those who have observed the acupuncturist in his native surroundings have noted that it is not used in children and that when used in surgery the level of analgesia produced by acupuncture is frequently enhanced by the liberal use of local anaesthetic drugs—especially for incisions of the skin which produce acute pain.

Culture and group influences upon the patient by his peers, together with careful training prior to operation, undoubtedly add enormously to whatever basic neurophysiological mechanisms are being activated by the acupuncture needle. Preliminary training, known as autogenic training, is a powerful procedure which involves rehearsal of the entire surgical procedure that will be performed in order to familiarise the patient with it and so reduce fear of the unknown. This is associated with up to two weeks training in relaxation techniques and is reinforced by discussions with patients who have been treated successfully. In this way the confidence of the patient and his motivation to go through surgery without pain is boosted to the highest levels.

Neurophysiological explanations for the effects of acupuncture are centred upon the view that the stimulus from the needle promotes the activation of pain inhibiting mechanisms in the central nervous system. The fact that many acupoints lie over or close to the paths of peripheral and cutaneous nerves supports the idea that direct stimulation of nerves is important, and the observation that there is often no correlation between the site of insertion of the needle and of the pain indicates that inhibition must occur at sites in the higher levels of the central nervous system. Recently it has been shown that an injection of a morphine antagonist, nalorphine, can reverse analgesia produced by acupuncture and this suggest that the latter may be causing the production of endogenous morphine-like substances such as enkephalins. Interestingly, hypnoanalgesia is not reversed by this drug and therefore the two methods of producing pain relief, though sharing the powerful psychological effects of suggestion and distraction, must differ to some extent in the physiological systems they activate.

To conclude, evidence taken from a large number of attempts to induce analgesia reveals that in Western medicine acupuncture has not proved very effective and that it is almost impossible to determine which patients will respond. Experimental studies reveal that only 10 to 15 per cent of patients requiring surgery develop adequate analgesia under its influence and therefore it is unsuitable for this purpose. However, there are reports of dramatic improvements amongst patients who suffer from migraine and some non-painful disorders. Therefore, as in the case of biofeedback, there is a need for continued careful study of the basis for, and effects of, acupuncture if it is to gain a permanent place in the range of treatments available to patients who suffer pain.

THE DEVELOPMENT AND FUNCTION OF CENTRES FOR PAIN RELIEF

The complexity of problems posed by patients with chronic pain, especially that which is due to a benign disorder, or which is caused solely or chiefly by psychological mechanisms, means that their investigation and treatment is likely to be most successful if carried out by a group of specialists with different skills in the treatment of pain. When first established the Pain Clinics were concerned chiefly with physical treatments, usually nerve blocking techniques performed by anaesthetists. In 1961 Dr Bonica (an anaesthetist) established the first multi-disciplinary clinic in Seattle, USA, and nowadays most clinics have specialists from anaesthetics, neurology, neurosurgery, psychiatry, psychology and radiotherapy, and sometimes from general practice, on their staff or easily available for consultation. As management virtually always involves far more than physical treatment and should encompass the patient's family, the team should include occupational and physiotherapists and a social worker. Most clinics in Britain fall short of this ideal and offer only a limited outpatient service, but the most highly developed, which are found in the United States and some European countries, lay emphasis upon the use of inpatient care in specialist centres.

Ideally, prior to admission to a treatment programme, all patients should be interviewed by a psychiatrist and undergo psychological tests designed to assess pain levels, personality and attitudes to health, and to search for evidence of formal emotional disturbances, such as anxiety or depressive neurosis and hypochondriasis. The results of the tests serve as a baseline for later assessments of the effectiveness of treatment. This part of a patient's assessment is often made a condition of entry to treatment in order to overcome the reluctance of many to be interviewed by a psychiatrist or a psychologist. If the treatment programme contains an element of behaviour therapy, the patient's behaviour will be assessed also—for example careful notes will be taken of requests for medicines, levels of activity, amounts of bed rest taken and evidence of manipulation of staff or patients in order to gain sympathy, avoid work or to obtain drugs.

A social worker is given the task of carrying out an assessment of the effect of the patient's illness upon the family and in turn the effect of the family's attitudes upon the patient. He or she also takes particular note of financial or housing difficulties and is on the lookout for signs of breakdown amongst family members.

Treatment must be under the direction of one person who is medically qualified. If the problem has a definite organic basis patients are usually in the care of a specialist surgeon, often a neurosurgeon, or a physician, and where the pain is primarily or solely generated by psychological factors, by a psychiatrist. Apart from the specialist treatment prescribed, nurses, physiotherapists and occupational therapists play an important part in both the physical care of the patient, which is regarded by most as their main role, and also in dealing with emotional difficulties too. As training in this area is often lacking amongst paramedical staff, case conferences and teaching seminars are used to ensure that they can fully appreciate and develop their respective roles. Psychologists play a key role in the treatment of patients by operant conditioning and receive help from nurses and other clinic staff who chart the various aspects of behaviour being modified. They also play an active part in helping patients to achieve their previously agreed treatment goals—which almost always include an increase in physical activity, a reduction in drugs for pain and an increase in social activities.

At the conclusion of intensive treatment the patient is discharged home and given further support over a period of months at an outpatient clinic and by home visits from the social worker. The latter's role is often that of helping the family and the patient to adjust to a state of chronic disability and also helping them to devise realistic goals in various areas of family life. The success or otherwise of the family in making the adjustments placed upon them by the patient's difficulties can be passed back to the physician in charge who, at his outpatient clinic, is unlikely to detect the more subtle difficulties that patients and their relatives encounter at home.

19

The treatment of pain in surgical patients

The prospect of having to undergo surgery is an unpleasant one for most people no matter how necessary it is or how much reassurance is given by family, friends, doctors and nurses. It is a situation from which there is little opportunity to escape, one which must be endured alone and one with a considerable element of the unknown in it. The patient must submit to the advice of the surgeon who is a highly regarded and trusted individual and who is generally treated by the patient with a degree of trust which has a childlike quality in its unquestioning dependency. The causes of patients' anxieties are not always expressed, and perhaps not even appreciated in any detail by them, the chief ones being having to experience pain, having to undergo an anaesthetic which is seen as the only part of the operation of which they will be aware, and anxiety about the outcome of treatment. Many patients are upset about being separated from their families and although in a ward where others share this experience they feel a sense of separation and loneliness, the depth of which is not always fully appreciated. Attempts to bridge the gulf between home and hospital are reflected in patients' collections of family photographs kept on the locker or bed table, often of their wedding if they are young, and of children or grandchildren when older.

Analysis of the underlying meanings of fears and other emotional experiences reveals that pain is not only regarded as a necessary part of the treatment by most, but in some instances it is seen as a punishment rightly or wrongly meted out to them. In clinical practice it is quite common for patients to ask why they should be ill and in pain when they live 'a good life', often comparing themselves with someone they know who has not done so and yet remains healthy. They may, as previously stated, talk about pain and the actual process of anaesthesia and surgery as a means of expressing a sense of anxiety about other less obvious issues, and prior to the operation itself this may well be about the question of whether or not it will be successful and restore them to good health. In the case of an anaesthetic, patients quite often fear losing their self-control and may wish to be reassured that the procedure is quite safe.

Looking at the way patients cope with pre-operative anxieties shows that there are three broad categories into which they may be grouped and the relation of these to post-operative behaviour is worth considering. The first pattern of coping is shown by patients who express an active fear of hospitals, surgery and everything associated with them. They shrink from operative treatment and avoid it if at all possible, coping poorly should it become necessary. Examination of such individuals usually reveals evidence of marked neurotic traits, especially proneness to anxiety, and perhaps a past history of a neurotic illness. By contrast with this group there is a second in which patients show little or no fear of surgery and, indeed, seem calm and quite relaxed being prepared for what is to come and expressing great confidence both in the surgeon, who in their opinion will be successful, and in their own ability to come through the treatment. They minimise the dangers and exude an air of confidence and invulnerability. They are often said to show an 'avoidance coping response'. These characteristics are obviously to the patient's advantage and will be a great asset when they have to cope with the post-operative stage of treatment. Indeed, such people appear to have fewer minor complications following surgery and this may be because they dismiss any symptoms that appear as trivial, or do not even mention them, whereas the first group mentioned would cope poorly with the same problems and demand a good deal of attention. However, this set of characteristics is not always helpful because there is evidence suggesting that individuals who normally cope in this way become hostile and resentful if serious complications develop. Thus, it is in cases where surgery is straightforward and likely to be successful that they cope well and inability to deal emotionally with serious complications seems to be related to the earlier denial of the fact that they could ever occur. In other words there is some benefit in anticipating what lies ahead and in rehearsing it mentally as part of building up a strategy for coping. Between these two extremes lies a third group of patients who are moderately fearful of what is to come but not overwhelmed by their feelings. They do not on the one hand deny anxiety and avoid asking questions, but seek information about all stages of the treatment thereby giving themselves a factual framework upon which to develop their emotional safeguards in advance.

Clearly, from what has been said it is important to know whether or not it is likely that a patient will experience moderate to severe pain after surgery if the doctor is to deal with one of his or her most pressing anxieties in the pre-operative phase. Most of our information about the painfulness of various disorders and their treatment has been passed down from one generation of doctors to the next in an informal manner. However, we have more specific methods of estimating the painfulness of illnesses, for example, by recording patients' needs for analgesic drugs post-operatively. Table 19 shows the requirements for them after different types of surgery and demonstrates that most pain is experienced after operations on parts of the body that are constantly moving, for example the chest or abdomen, whereas operations upon the head and neck are less painful although they are quite sensitive areas.

Table 19 The severity of post-operative pain as reflected in patients needs for analgesic drugs

Surgical procedure	% Patients requiring analgesics
General surgery (all kinds)	74
Biliary surgery	95
Thoracotomy	75
Appendicectomy	75
Hernia repair	25
Scrotal surgery	2
Operations on the head and neck	15–50

The treatment of post-operative pain requires attention to the patient's physical and psychological needs which are closely allied to each other. Physical suffering includes the experience of pain and also the effects of fatigue, sleeplessness and other unpleasant physical symptoms, such as nausea and vomiting, together with the effects of immobility or uncomfortable postures due to the presence of surgical dressings, appliances, intravenous infusions, monitors and the other paraphernalia of modern surgery. The atmosphere of the recovery room, or intensive care ward, is usually totally strange to the patient, who was almost certainly in a general ward beforehand. This places yet another stress upon him and calls for fresh powers to cope with the anxieties provoked. All these factors, which are present to a variable extent after surgery, tend to heighten fear and loneliness and to increase patients' dependence on medical and nursing staff who have been invested already with powers which stem both from the patient's past experience of doctors and hospitals, and a phantasy life freely fed by newspapers, magazines and television programmes. Medical staff and nurses are regarded as being in control and if the patient is given warm emotional support his or her vision of the staff's role in care is fulfilled and a sense of security is established. If, however, doctors or nurses give most of their attention to the practicalities of managing equipment, or remain aloof and distant, especially if any form of post-operative complication develops, patients begin to develop a sense of anxiety, tension and even hostility, which has an important effect upon their ability to cope, reflected both in pain levels and demands for pain-relieving drugs.

The practical matter of prescribing pain-relieving drugs has been subjected to considerable research and aspects of this to be taken into consideration include the relationship between pre-operative levels of fear and anxiety and post-operative pain, the value of preoperative physical and psychological preparation, and the prescription of analgesic drugs following operation. Although the relationship between pre-operative levels of anxiety and post-operative pain is not as close as might be expected, it is generally agreed that pre-operative preparation of patients for surgery involving discussion of the procedures to be carried out and postoperative difficulties they may well encounter with the surgeon and anaesthetist who will be involved, is to be recommended. Pre-operative measures designed to teach patients how to relax, to breathe and to position themselves correctly after surgery have been found to improve a patient's confidence and to halve the need for analgesics postoperatively. Premedication is a routine which reduces anxiety and fear immediately before surgery and this is of considerable benefit especially to those who show very high levels of pre-operative

Table 20 Relief of post-operative pain by analgesic drugs. Patients' rating of drug potencies (from Morrison, Loan & Dundee (1971) *British Medical Journal*, Vol. 3, pp. 287–290, with permission)

Degree of relief	Analgesic drugs	
More than 80% pain relief	Diamorphine	5 mg
	Papaveretum	20 mg
	Oxycodone	10 mg
	Levorphanol	2 mg
	Pethidine	100 mg
	Methadone	10 mg
	Morphine 10 mg + Cyclizine 50 mg (Cyclimorph 10)	
75–80% pain relief	Morphine	10 gm
	Pentazocine	20 mg
	Phenoperidine	2 mg
	Pethidine 100 mg + Levallorphan 1.25 mg (Pethilorfan 100	
70–74% pain relief	Dextromoramide	5 mg
50–69% pain relief	Dihydrocodeine	50 mg
	Fentanyl	0.2 mg
	Phenazocine	2 mg
Less than 50% pain relief	Saline	

Table 21 Patients' opinions about the efficacy of analgesic drugs taking account of pain relief and side-effects experienced (From Morrison, Loan & Dundee (1971) *British Medical Journal*, Vol 3, pp. 287–290, with permission.)

Percentage of patients reporting 'successful' pain relief	Analgesic drugs	
More than 75	Levorphanol	2 mg
70–75	Morphine 10 mg + Cyclizine 50 mg (Cyclimorph 10)	
	Oxycodone	10 mg
	Pentazocine	20 mg
65–69	Methadone	10 mg
	Papaveretum	20 mg
60–64	Diamorphine	5 mg
	Morphine	10 mg
	Pentazocine	40 mg
55–59	Dextromoramide	5 mg
	Morphine	15 mg
50–55	Fentanyl	0.2 mg
	Pethidine	100 mg
Less than 50	Dihydrocodeine	50 mg
	Pethidine 100 mg + Levallorphan 1.25 mg (Pethilorfan 100)	
	Phenazocine	2 mg

tension. The use of an opiate in this situation not only helps in this respect but also reduces the immediate need for pain-relieving drugs after surgery.

Postoperative medication and its timing is influenced by the anaesthetic agent used during surgery. For example, tricholoroethylene has an analgesic effect and is associated with a delay in the need for analgesics and a reduction in the doses of them required post-operatively. Thirteen drugs commonly used as post-operative medication were studied by Doctors Morrison, Loan and Dundee, and their effectiveness in controlling pain in 740 patients who underwent either upper or lower abdominal operations, that is those which are regarded as amongst the most painful patients have to endure, are shown in Tables 20 and 21. Table 20 shows patients' estimates of the efficiency of drugs in relieving pain. The analgesics have been ranked according to the degree of pain relief gained from them. The investigators were also able to rank the drugs according to their 'overall success' with patients which involved taking account of their potency and any tendency to produce respiratory depression and/or impairment of consciousness (Table 21). Levorphanol was ranked first because, when compared with morphine, it produced less drowsiness. It was also noticed that larger doses of morphine and pentazocine were less acceptable than smaller ones, reinforcing the point that provision of the optimum dose of the drug should be the aim of the prescriber, therefore he should achieve maximum pain relief with minimum side effects. Single agents are preferable to drug combinations. In the study mentioned only in the case of cyclimorph '10' (morphine 10 mg, cyclizine 50 mg) did there appear to be potentiation of the effect of the analgesic member of the pair and this may have been due to the reduction of the side effects of morphine by cyclizine which does not have analgesic properties of its own. By comparison, in the case of pethilorphan 100 (pethidine 100 mg, levallorphan 1.25 mg), the potency of pethidine was reduced by the presence of the other drug. To conclude, the efficacy of a range of the commonly used analgesics recommended for the control of different levels of post-operative pain is given in Tables 20 and 21 and general rules governing their administration can be found on page 164.

The reader will have noticed that the studies mentioned concern only analgesics of moderate or high potency and that they were administered by intramuscular injection for pain caused by abdominal surgery. This may give the impression that the use of moderate to powerful analgesics by injection is the only way of dealing with post-operative pain. This is far from the truth. Wherever possible analgesics should be given by mouth, sublingually or rectally, and

Table 22 Post-operative pain management (After Clarke, I. M. C. and Budd, K. with permission)

Route of administration	Drug	Dose	Frequency (hours)
Analgesics for mild to moderate pain			
Oral	Paracetamol	1 g	4
	Codeine phosphate	60 mg	4
	Soluble Aspirin	300–600 mg	4
	Any simple combination		
Analgesics for moderate to severe pain			
Oral	*Papaveretum 10 mg	20 mg	4
	Diamorphine 10 mg	10–20 mg	4
Sublingual	Phenazocine 5 mg	5 mg (max 20 mg)	4–6
	*Buprenorphine 0.2 mg	0.2–0.4 mg	6–8
Rectal	Morphine supps. 30 mg	30–60 mg	6
	Oxycodone 30 mg	30–60 mg	6–10
IM/IV	Morphine	10–20 mg	
	Diamorphine	5–10 mg	4–6
	Papaveretum	10–20 mg	
	*Buprenorphine	0.3–0.6 mg	6–8

* These analgesics are *not* controlled drugs

the strength of an analgesic should be related to the level of pain a patient suffers in the post-operative period. Thus injections should be given only where patients are not fully conscious or troubled by vomiting. A simple guide to the use of analgesics for post-operative pain has been prepared by two anaesthetists, Drs I. M. C. Clarke and K. Budd, and it is given in Table 22.

20

Pain and emotion in malignant disease

Pain in malignant disease brings concern about its cause, likely duration and its intensity. Many patients and their relatives believe pain to be an inevitable part of this type of illness, although half those patients who have a malignant disease are pain-free. It appears that approximately a third experience unrelieved pain, however, with skilled management this figure can be reduced substantially. For example, two thirds of the patients admitted to St Christoper's Hospice in London between 1972 and 1977 had serious pain problems and sought treatment there for this reason. After careful assessment and treatment only 1 per cent were left with pain that remained difficult to control. The pain is usually chronic but fluctuates in its severity, being influenced by many factors, some physical and some psychological. Amongst the latter feelings of helplessness and futility which appear as the disease progresses make it difficult to tolerate pain, which in itself seems to have no purpose and which one might call 'useless pain'. As a result patients become demoralised and feel isolated in their suffering. Specific anxieties about being separated from the family and friends, loss of work and life's goals, the consequences of the illness for others, increasing dependency, losing one's faculties, mutilation and death are all potential sources of tension and depression. In these circumstances care must be taken not to increase a patient's miseries by prescribing analgesic drugs in very high doses and at levels where their toxic effects become objectionable. Anorexia, nausea, vomiting, reduced powers of concentration, and a lowered level of consciousness are uncomfortable and unwanted and it is far better that the doctor should move on to a drug of greater potency and use it in a low dose, thereby keeping pain at bay and drug toxicity to a minimum.

Patients with cancer are said to pass through four stages in their emotional responses to a progressive and ultimately fatal illness; stages which relatives pass through too though not necessarily at the same time. The author's view is that the reactions described may or may not occur and the order in which they do so differs from person to person. Initially the patient may exhibit denial, a mental mechanism which in this case protects against the likelihood of overwhelming anxiety based on a fear of death. Next may come anger—'why should it happen to me' is the cry, and blame may be laid upon the patient by himself, or upon others. He or she then accepts the diagnosis, but looks to the doctor to cure the disease and when therapeutic measures are seen to fail depression occurs and may be sufficiently intense to lead to suicide, especially amongst older, single or widowed men. Finally, patients accept that death is inevitable and come to terms with the prospect in many cases, in some with resignation and sadness, and in others with cheerfulness and determination to be active to their life's end. In the stages where the patient has not yet come to terms with the prospect of dying complaints of physical symptoms, including pain, and demands for treatment may be high, acting as a way of coping with underlying tension and communicating this to others. Depression may present with complaints of intolerable pain as the patient feels helpless in the grip of the disease and sometimes feels deserted by doctors and deceived by family and friends. For some doctors the failure of the patient to respond to their treatment may lead to loss of interest which may be due either to a feeling of inability to cope with the patient's questions about their illness, especially enquiries about its outcome, or because of their own inability to cope with the fact that they have not yet learned to accept failure to respond to one kind of treatment does not mean that they should not pursue other lines, especially when these are basically psychological. For example, when dealing with patients in pain in the last stages of their lives doctors who let a patient know that they will not be deserted and demonstrate this by regular visits, by sitting with them for a few minutes each day will provide a great deal of comfort and security through the sense of warmth and support this brings. Coupled with appropriate physical treatment this approach has a great deal to commend it as a means of reducing suffering and pain.

The relationship of patients to their relatives is disturbed by the illness and knowledge of it produces in the latter anxiety, fear and even horror or disgust. It also brings worries about coping with their own fears of death and here the doctor's understanding and support is also needed. In Britain the diagnosis of cancer is often withheld from the patient bringing a good deal of anguish to the relatives who either wish to avoid the full implications of the diagnosis themselves as part of their process of coming to terms with the problem, or who wish to conform with the doctor's view. In either case their behaviour and comments soon confirm suspicions in the patient's mind yet binds them in a 'conspiracy of silence'. In fact about three quarters of those who will die within six months are aware that this will happen, but the tension aroused by the way in which the issue is handled may lead to increasing demands for attention, bouts of hostility and requests for medication for a variety of physical symptoms. Relatives may experience guilt as part of their reaction to the threat of loss of their wife, husband or child and, as a result, project their own feelings upon others, blaming them for what has happened or, in the case of doctors and nurses, for failure to effect a cure. Alternatively, they may become depressed or develop pain of a similar kind to that experienced by the sick person.

The physical treatment of pain in malignant disease depends upon its cause and site of origin. For example, pain is often relatively easily remedied if due to infection, constipation or pressure sores, whereas it is more difficult to control when it is due to tumour invading sensitive tissues such as bone or nerve. Thus, in addition to the use of analgesics, the doctor may prescribe, according to the conditions, antibiotics, anti-inflammatory drugs or cytotoxic drugs. He may advise the use of irradiation, nerve blocks, cordotomy, or hypophysectomy, together with simple measures such as immobilisation of the limbs or local heat. These, together with measures to reduce a patient's self-concern or boredom by increasing activity and interest through encouragement to read papers or books, to watch television and to attend occupational therapy groups, or to make conversation with other patients and visitors, markedly improves an individual's ability to cope with pain.

ANALGESIC DRUGS

There are two main classes of drugs available. The non-narcotics which are used for mild to moderate pain, and the narcotics or methadone derivatives for moderate to severe pain. The drugs of choice are as follows:

1. *Non-narcotics*. These include aspirin, paracetamol, and non-steroidal anti-inflammatory drugs such as diflunisal or indomethacin (Dolobid or Indocid).
2. *Narcotics or methadone derivatives*. These include morphine, diamorphine, phenazocine, buprenorphine, dextropropoxyphene with paracetamol or aspirin (Distalgesic or Napsalgesic), dextromoramide, dipipanone, dihydrocodeine and codeine.

ADMINISTRATION OF DRUGS

Drugs may be given by mouth, parenterally or contained in a suppository, and in all cases should be given regularly rather than on demand.

Administration by mouth

From the patient's and doctor's point of view alike this is the most convenient and acceptable method of treatment and should be used as long as possible. Non-narcotics and narcotics may both be given by this route, the contra-indication being persistent nausea and vomiting uncontrolled by anti-emetics. A number of patients are unable to tolerate aspirin and it is not prescribed where there is a history of peptic ulceration as alternatives, e.g. paracetamol or benorylate, are available. By contrast some individuals have a high level of tolerance for the drug and in a 600 mg dose it is approximately equal in potency to 65 mg of dextropropoxyphene. Doses of 1200 mg four-hourly may be used with good effect where a smaller dose gives inadequate relief. Pentazocine (Fortral), is only one-third as effective by mouth when compared with an injection and, as it has the potency of two tablets of dextropropoxyphene in an oral dose of 50 mg and has significant psychomimetic effects, the latter is preferred. Dextropropoxyphene alone is a very mild analgesic and less potent than codeine, therefore it is almost always given in a compound tablet with paracetamol or aspirin. Pethidine is also less effective by mouth than by injection and, as its duration of action is short, being two to three hours only, it is more suitable for acute than for chronic pain. Oxycodone pectinate (Proladone) in a dose of 10 to 15 mg and codeine phosphate 15 mg, each give four to five hours of analgesia and are as effective by mouth or by injection. The former may also be given in a suppository in a dose of 30 mg six-to eight-hourly which is especially useful for night time as it can be given in the late evening to cover the hours of sleep.

If the level of pain increases beyond the control of drugs mentioned, it is advisable that a more powerful narcotic compound be used. Dipipanone with cyclizine (Diconal) is recommended in this situation in a dose of 1 to 2 tablets four-to six-hourly.

Even the most powerful narcotics may be taken by mouth and over a wide dose range which permits control of moderately severe but unchanging chronic pain or, by means of steadily increasing doses, pain of increasing intensity. For example, both morphine and diamorphine may be given in doses ranging from 5 mg to 10 mg and an upper dose level not exceeding 30 mg of either drug is adequate for most patients.

Morphine and codeine may be given in the form of an elixir, known as Brompton Cocktail, also containing cocaine, or cocaine and chlorpromazine. This is one example:

Morphine hydrochloride	5 mg
Cocaine hydrochloride	5 mg/m ml
Ethyl alcohol	95% B.P., 2.5 ml
Syrup (66% sucrose in water W/V)	5 ml
Chloroform water	220 ml

The dose range of this elixir is 2.5 to 10 ml, and alternative forms containing morphine are given in the British National Formulary. In recent years studies carried out at Hospices for the terminally ill have shown that a simpler oral preparation of morphine or diamorphine is preferable to the traditional Brompton Elixir. The use of a single narcotic analgesic permits an accurate dose to be administered. Also cocaine is omitted because it is expensive, and because it causes drowsiness which is disliked by some patients. The solution consists of morphine or diamorphine (5 mg) in water or chloroform water (5 ml) with added flavouring.

Parenteral administration

For many patients only in the last hours of life need narcotics such as diamorphine be given parenterally and then in doses which are half those given by mouth. This drug is preferred to morphine at this stage because with its greater solubility it may be given in larger doses. At times drugs have to be given parenterally earlier in the illness because gastro-intestinal complications prevent patients taking them by mouth.

THE SIDE EFFECTS OF TREATMENT

Nausea and vomiting are troublesome and unpleasant symptoms which narcotics may exacerbate or cause themselves, especially if patients are up and about. Anti-emetics are required in these circumstances and those most often used are the phenothiazines, for example prochlorperazine (Stemetil) in a dose starting at 5 mg, and chlorpromazine (Largactil) in a dose starting at 12.5 mg, each being given at the same time as the chosen analgesic. These drugs have the added advantage of producing a degree of tranquillisation, they are also antipsychotic, and chlorpromazine potentiates analgesics in doses of 25 mg or more. However, the latter may also precipitate or increase feelings of depression which, if severe, require antidepressant drug therapy. Where nausea and vomiting are not particularly troublesome but excessive emotional tension is present, minor tranquillisers may be used as an alternative. Other side effects of narcotics which cause difficulties are constipation, drowsiness and drug dependence. Constipation may be countered by the use of stool softeners and laxatives to reduce the possibilities of faecal impaction. The development of drowsiness seems to vary from one individual to another, but often clears within three to four days of beginning drug therapy. Tolerance and drug dependence are encountered, but where narcotics are given in the manner described with other supportive measures, both physical and psychological, tolerance is seldom a problem and physical dependency, which is much more common than psychological dependency and which takes two to three weeks to develop, may be eliminated if necessary by gradual reduction in the dose of the drug and the use of other measures for pain relief.

GUIDELINES ON THE USE OF DRUGS FOR THE CONTROL OF PAIN IN ADULT PATIENTS WITH CANCER

Mild pain

A significant number of cancer patients experience only mild pain and many who have severe pain had mild to moderate pain earlier in their illnesses. Therefore, the use of a non-narcotic analgesic of relatively low potency is often indicated. Those commonly prescribed are:

Aspirin. Dose: soluble aspirin 300–1200 mg four to six hourly.

Paracetamol (e.g. Panadol). Dose: 1 g four to six hourly.

Dextropropoxyphene hydrochloride 32.5 mg with paracetamol 325 mg (Distalgesic). Dose: 1–2 tablets four to six hourly.

Dextropropoxyphene napsylate 50 mg (equivalent to 32.5 mg of hydrochloride) with aspirin 500 mg (Napsalgesic). Dose: 1–2 tablets four to six hourly.

For pain arising from bone:

Diflunisal (Dolobid). Dose: 250–500 mg twice daily. This is a long-acting, non-corticosteroidal, anti-inflammatory drug.

Moderate pain

Replace non-narcotic drugs with weaker narcotic analgesics or those from the methadone group.

Codeine phosphate. Dose: 10–60 mg four to six hourly.

Codeine phosphate 8 mg with aspirin 500 mg (Codis). Dose: 1–2 soluble tablets four to six hourly.
Dihydrocodeine phosphate (DF-118). Dose: 30 mg tablets four to six hourly. Elixir (10 mg in 5 ml). Dose: 5–15 ml four to six hourly.
Dihydrocodeine tartrate 10 mg with paracetamol 500 mg (Paramol-118). Dose: 1 tablet four hourly to 2 tablets six hourly. Compounds containing DF-118 should be taken after meals.
Dipipanone hydrochloride 10 mg with cyclizine 30 mg (Diconal). Dose: 1 tablet four to six hourly initially.
Dextromoramide tartrate (Palfium). Dose: 10 mg four to six hourly initially. This is a short-acting analgesic which is often used as 'top-up' for bouts of acute or chronic pain.
Oral morphine 5–10 mg in solution. Dose: 5–10 mg six hourly for maintenance.

Severe pain

Initially use oral narcotics on a regular basis to obtain constant blood levels and to prevent pain 'breaking through' the analgesic barrier.
Oral morphine. Dose: 5–90 mg four to six hourly. Patients seldom need a dose greater than 30 mg. The maximum effective dose is 90 mg.
Oral diamorphine. Dose: 5–100 mg four to six hourly. Patients seldom need a dose greater than 30 mg. Oral diamorphine is 1½ times more potent than oral morphine.
Morphine suppositories. Dose: 15–30 mg/supp., 1–2 supp. six hourly.
Oxycodone suppositories. Dose: 30 mg, 1–2 supp. eight hourly or at bedtime.

Alternatives to morphine and diamorphine

Phenazocine hydrobromide (Narphen). Doses: 5 mg four to six hourly. 5 mg of phenazocine is equivalent to 25 mg of morphine. The maximum recommended dose is 20 mg. This drug is available in oral and sublingual forms.
Buprenorphine hydrochloride (Temgesic). Dose: 0.2–0.4 mg six to eight hourly. The tablets are dissolved under the tongue.

Injections of narcotic analgesics for severe pain

Morphine sulphate. Dose: 10–20 mg four to six hourly.
Diamorphine. Dose: 5–10 mg four to six hourly.
Micro-crystalline morphine suspension (Duromorph). Dose: (64 mg/ml), 32 mg two or three times daily. The dose depends upon previous doses of oral morphine. For example, 32 mg of Duromorph (0.5 ml)

twice daily is equivalent to 30 mg of oral morphine five to six times daily.

Buprenorphine hydrochloride (Temgesic). Dose: (0.3 mg/ml), 0.3–0.6 mg six to eight hourly.

CONTROL OF NAUSEA AND VOMITING

Occasionally anti-emetics are required by patients taking narcotic analgesics, especially if they are ambulant. The following drugs are used:

Prochlorperazine (Stemetil). Doses: I.M. 12.5–25 mg eight hourly. Review the need for an anti-emetic every two or three days and transfer to an oral or rectal form as soon as possible (5–20 mg by mouth to a maximum of 30 mg in 24 hours).

Metoclopramide (Maxolon). Dose: I.M. 10 mg eight hourly. Change to the oral form if possible; up to 10 mg eight hourly by mouth.

Cyclizine (Valoid). Doses: I.M. 50 mg eight hourly. Change to the oral form if possible; 50 mg eight hourly.

MANAGEMENT OF CONSTIPATION

In view of the tendency of narcotic analgesics to cause constipation it is advisable to prescribe a stool softener and bowel stimulant, e.g.

Danthron 25 mg and poloxamer '188' (Dorbanex). Dose: (200 mg per 5 ml). 5–10 ml at night.

Danthron 75 mg and poloxamer '188' (Dorbanex Forte). Dose: (1 g per 5 ml). 5 ml at night. Adjust the dose according to each patient's needs.

Bibliography

REFERENCES

The full references to the works of interest quoted in the text are as follows:

Bonica, J. J. (1977) Basic principles in managing chronic pain. *Archives of Surgery*, Vol. 112, pp. 783–788, (This paper deals with the management of a pain clinic.)

Dalessio, D. J. (ed.) (1980) *Wolff's Headache and other head pains*. Oxford: Oxford University Press.

Engel, G. L. (1959) 'Psychogenic' pain and the pain-prone patient. *American Journal of Medicine*, Vol. 26, pp. 899–918.

Eysenck, H. & Eysenck, S. G. B. (1964) *Manual of the Eysenck Personality Inventory*. University of London Press.

Fordyce, W. E., Fowler, R. S. & Delateur, B. (1968) An application of behaviour modification techniques to a problem of chronic pain. *Behaviour Research and Therapy*, Vol. 6, pp. 105–107.

Hilton, J. (1863) *Lectures on Rest and Pain*. London: Bell.

Keele, K. D. (1957) *Anatomies of Pain*. Oxford: Blackwell Scientific (An historical reference)

Lewis, T. (1942) *Pain*. New York: The Macmillan Company (An historical reference)

Melzack, R. (1973) *The Puzzle of Pain*. Ch. 6. Harmondsworth: Penguin.

Melzack, R. (1975) The McGill Pain Questionnaire: major properties and scoring methods. *Pain*, **1**, 277–299.

Melzack, R. & Wall, P. D. (1965) Pain mechanisms: a new theory. *Science*, **150**, 971.

Morrison, J. D., Loan, W. B. & Dundee, J. W. (1971) Controlled comparison of the efficacy of fourteen preparations in the relief of post-operative pain. *British Medical Journal*, Vol. 3, pp. 287–290.

Pain glossary. (1979) *Pain*, **6**, 249–252.

Sternbach, R. A., Murphy, R. W., Timmermans, G., Greenhoot, J. H. & Akeson, W. H. (1974) Measuring the severity of clinical pain. In *An International Symposium on Pain*. Ed. Bonica, J. J. *Advances in Neurology*, Vol. 4, pp. 281–288. New York: Raven Press.

Szasz, J. S. (1968) The psychology of persistent pain. A portrait of L'Homme Douloureux. In *Pain, Proceedings of An International Symposium on Pain*. Ed. Soulairac, H., Cahn, J. & Charpentier, J. pp. 93–113. New York: Academic Press.

Waddell, G., McCulloch, J. A., Kummel, E. & Venner, R. M. (1980) Non-organic physical signs in low-back pain. *Spine*, 5, 117–125.

FURTHER READING

The following texts are recommended for further reading;

Anatomy and physiology of the nervous system

Bowsher, D. (1975) *Introduction to the Anatomy and Physiology of The Nervous System*, 3rd ed. Oxford: Blackwell.

Melzack, R. (1973) *The Puzzle of Pain*. Harmondsworth: Penguin.

Sternbach R. A. (1968). *Pain. A Psychophysiological Analysis*. New York: Academic Press.

Psychosocial aspects of pain

Kosterlitz, H. W., Terenius, L. Y. (eds) (1980) *Pain and Society*. Report of the Dahlem Workshop on Pain and Society. Verlag Chemie: Weinheim, Deerfield Beach, Florida, Basel.

Merskey, H. & Spear, F. G. (1967) *Pain. Psychological and Psychiatric Aspects*. London: Bailliére Tindall and Cassell.

Sternbach, R. A. (1974) *Pain Patients, Traits and Treatments*. New York: Academic Press.

Sternbach, R. A. (ed.) (1978) *The Psychology of Pain*. New York: Raven Press.

Treatment of pain

Balint, M. (1964) *The Doctor, His Patient and The Illness*. 2nd edn. London: Pitman.

Lipton, S. (1979) Relief of pain in clinical practice. Oxford: Blackwell Scientific (Physical methods of pain relief)

Roy, R., & Tunks, E. (eds.) (1982) *Chronic pain. Psychosocial factors in rehabilitation*. Baltimore: Williams and Wilkins.

Silverstone T. & Turner P. (1974) *Drug Treatment in Psychiatry*. London: Routledge & Kegan Paul.

Glossary

Medicines mentioned in the text are listed alphabetically under their approved names, with their British and U.S. equivalents.

British approved name	British proprietary name	U.S. approved name	U.S. proprietary name
Acetazolamide	Diamox, Sustets	Acetazolamide	Hydrazol
Amethocaine hydrochloride		Tetracaine hydrochloride	Pontocaine
Amitriptyline B.P.	Amizol Domical Lentizol Limbritol-10 Saroten Triptafen-DA Triptafen-Minor Triptafen-Forte Tryptizol		Elavil Endap
Amphetamine Sulph. B.P. (Controlled drug)	Benzedrine		Raphetamine
Aspirin B.P. B.N.F. (Acetylsalicylic acid)	Angiers Junior Aspirin Asagran Aspergum Aspro Breoprin Caprin Chu-Pax Disprin and Junior Disprin Genasprin Levius Nuseals (Enteric sealed) Solprin	Aspirin capsules USNF	ASA Measurin
with codeine	Codis		
with codeine salicylamide phenolphthalein	Anodyne		
with caffeine			

British approved name	British proprietary name	U.S. approved name	U.S. proprietary name
with paracetamol codeine	Veganin		
with codeine caffeine phenolphthalein	'Hypon'		
with aminoacetic acid	Paynocil		
with paracetamol	Safapryn (Enteric coated)		
with butobarbitone	Tercin	Tercin	
with codeine phosphate caffeine citrate	Antoin		
Atropine sulphate			
Azapropazone	Rheumox		
Bamethan sulphate	Vasculit		
Benorylate	Benoral		
Bupivicaine hydrochloride	Marcain (with adrenaline) Marcain plain		
Buprenorphine	Temgesic		
Caffeine	See compound Aspirin tablets		
*Cannabis			
Carbamazepine B.P.	Tegretol		Tegretol
Chlordiazepoxide	Calmoden Librium Tropium		Librium Libritabs
Chlorpromazine B.P.	Chloractil Largactil		Chlor-PZ Promachel Promachlor Promapar Thoradex Thorazine
with amylobarbitone	Amargyl		
Cimetidine	Tagamet		
Clomipramine hydrochloride	Anafranil		
Cocaine			
Codeine Phosphate B.P. tablets			
Cyclizine hydrochloride	Marzine Valoid	Cyclizine	Marezine
Danthron poloxamer 188	Dorbanex Dorbanex Forte		
Dextromoramide tartrate	Palfium		
Dextropropoxyphene	Depronal SA Doloxene		Darvon Dolene

British approved name	British proprietary name	U.S. approved name	U.S. proprietary name
	SK65		Dolocap Mardon Propoxychel Proxagesic
with paracetamol	Distalgesic		
with aspirin	Dolasan		
with aspirin	Napsalgesic		
with amylobarbitone	Doloxytal		
Diamorphine hydrochloride	Heroin		
Diazepam B.P.	Atensine Tensium Valium		Valium
Diflunisal	Dolobid		
Dihydrocodeine tartrate B.P.	D.F. 118		
with aspirin	Onadox-118		
with paracetamol	Paramol-118		
Dipipanone hydrochloride	Diconal		
Droperidol	Proleptan	Droperidol	Inapsine
Ergotamine tartrate	Femergin Lingraine Medihaler-ergotamine	Ergotamine tartrate and caffeine tablets	Ergomar
with caffeine	Cafergot Effergot		
with cyclizine	Migril		
Eserine (see physostigmine)			
Ethoheptazine citrate			Zactame
with paracetamol	Zactipar		
with aspirin	Zactirin		
calcium carbonate			
with meprobamate aspirin calcium carbonate	Equagesic		
Fenoprofen	Fenopron		
Fentanyl citrate	Sublimaze	Fentanyl citrate Inj (U.S.P.)	
with droperidol	Thalamonal Injection		Innovar
Feprazone	Methrazone		
Flufenamic acid	Meralen		
Fluphenazine hydrochloride	Motival		
with nortriptyline			
Flurazepam	Dalmane	Flurazepam hydrochloride	

British approved name	British proprietary name	U.S. approved name	U.S. proprietary name
		capsules (USNF)	
Glyceryl trinitrate	Sustac Nitrocontin		Nitora Nitro-Bid Nitrolar Nitroprn Nitro-SA Nitrospan Nitroglya Nitrol Nitrostat Nitrong Nitrolex T.D.
with ethylmorphine hydrochloride hyoscyamine hydrochloride	Natirose		
with caffeine hydrobromide digitalis strophanthus tincture	Cardial Dellipsoids D18		
Ibuprofen	Brufen		
Idoxuridine Eyedrops	Kerecid Ophthalmadine	Idoxuridine ophthalmic solution	Stoxil
Imipramine	Berkomine Co-Caps Imipramine Dimipressin Norpramine Oppanyl Praminil Tofranil		Imavate Janimine Presamine SK-Pramine
Indomethacin	Imbrilon Indocid		Indocin
Ispaghula Husk	Fybogel Isogel		
Levorphanol tartrate	Dromoran		Levo-Dromoran
Lignocaine hydrochloride	Xylocaine Xylocard Lignostab	Lidocaine hydrochloride	Anestacon Lida-mantle
Lorazepam	Ativan		
*Lysergic acid			
Mebeverine hydrochloride	Colofac		
Medazepam	Nobrium		
Mefenamic acid	Ponstan		Ponstel
Meprobamate	Equanil Mepavlon		Amosene Kessobamate

British approved name	British proprietary name	U.S. approved name	U.S. proprietary name
	Meprate		Mepriam
	Milonorm		Meprotabs
	Miltown		Protran
	Miltown S-R		Qidbamate
	Tised		SK-Bamate
			Vio-Bamate
			Meprospan
with bendrofluazide	Tenavoid		
*Mescaline			
Methadone hydrochloride	Physeptone		Dolophine hydrochloride
			Westadone
Methysergide	Deseril		
Metoclopropamide	Maxolon		
Mianserin hydrochloride	Bolvidon		
	Norval		
Morphine sulphate injection			
Morphine microcrystalline suspension	Duromorph		
Morphine with cyclizine	Cyclimorph		
Naftidrofuryl oxalate	Praxilene		
Naloxone	Narcan		Narcan
Naproxen	Naprosyn		
Nitrazepam	Nitrazepam tablets		
	Mogadon		
	Remnos		
Opium	Nepenthe		
Oxazepam	Oxazepam capsules		Serax
	Oxazepam tablets		
	Serenid Forte		
	Serenid D		
Oxycodone pectinate	Proladone		Percodan
Oxyphenbutazone	Tandacote		Oxalid
with paracetamol	Tandalgesic		Tandearil
with aluminium hydroxide magnesium trisilicate	Tanderil-Alka		
Paracetamol	Calpol		Anuphen
	Pamol		Apamide
	Panadol		Capital
	Panadol soluble		Cen-Apap
	Panasorb		Dolanex
	Salzone		Febrigesic
	Ticelgesic		Febrogesic
			Korum

British approved name	British proprietary name	U.S. approved name	U.S. proprietary name
			Liquiprin
			Lyteca
			Nebs
			Neopap
			Phendex
			Proval
			SK-Apap
			Tapar
			Temlo
			Tempra
			Tylenol
			Valadol
with codeine phosphate butobarbitone	Budale		
with caffeine citrate	Cafadol		
with diphenhydramine hydrochloride ephedrine caffeine	Dolvan		
with chlormezanone	Lobak		
with codeine phosphate phenolphthalein	Medocodene		
with codeine phosphate	Neurodyne Caps.		
with orphenadrine citrate	Norgesic		
with codeine phosphate in Sorbitol basis	Panadeine Co		
with codeine phosphate 8 mg equivalent 1.5 g sodium citrate	Paracodol		
with codeine phosphate phenolphthalein	Paradeine		
with caffeine codeine phosphate phenolphthalein	Parahypon tablets		
with codeine phosphate	Parake		
with codeine phosphate caffeine	Paralgin tablets		
with codeine phosphate caffeine hydrate	Pardale		
with caffeine meprobamate	Paxidal		

British approved name	British proprietary name	U.S. approved name	U.S. proprietary name
Paracetamol (continued)			
with codeine phosphate caffeine in Sorbitol basis	Solpadeine		
Papaveratum and Hyoscine	Omnopon-Scopolamine		Pantopon
Pentazocine	Fortral		Talwin
with paracetamol	Fortagesic		
Pericyazine	Neulactil		
Perphenazine	Fentazin	Perphenazine	Trilafon
Pethidine hydrochloride	Pethidine Roche		Demerol
with promethazine hydrochloride	Pamergan P100 or Pamergan AP100/25		
with levallorphan tartrate	Pethilorfan		
†Phenacetin	Phenacetin tablets		Phenacetin
with caffeine	Phenacetin and Caffeine tablets		
with aspirin	Aspirin and Phenactin tablets		
with aspirin codeine phosphate	A.P.C. tablets		
	(Soluble A.P.C. tabs also available)		
Phenazocine hydrobromide	Narphen		
Phenelzine	Nardil		
Phenoperidine	Operidine		
Phenoxybenzamine	Phenoxybenzamine caps. Dibenyline		Dibenzyline
Phenylbutazone	Butacote Butazolidin Butazone Ethibute Flexazone Oppazone Tetnor		Azolid
with dried aluminium hydroxide gel magnesium trisilicate	Butazolidin Alka		

British approved name	British proprietary name	U.S. approved name	U.S. proprietary name
with prednisone	Delta-Butazolidin		
with paracetamol	Parazolidin		
Phenytoin	Epanutin	Phenytoin	Dilatin Dilabid Ekko Kessodanten
Physostigmine salicylate or sulphate		Physostigmine salicylate	Antilirium Isopto eserine
Pilocarpine hydrochloride	Isopto-carpine	Pilocarpine hydrochloride	Adsorbocarpine Mi-Pilo Mistura P Pilocar
Potassium chlorazepate	Tranxene		
Prilocaine hydrochloride	Citanest Citanest with adrenaline	Prilocaine hydrochloride	
Prochlorperazine mesylate	Stemetil		
Propantheline bromide	Pro-banthine		
*Psilocybin			
Ranitidine	Zantac		
Sulphasalazine	Salazopyrin		
Temazepam	Normison		
Trichlorethylene	Triklone Trilene		
Zimelidine	Zelmid		

† Prescription of these medicines not recommended in view of the nephrotoxic effects of phenacetin.

* It is unlawful to possess these drugs under schedule IV of Misuse of Drugs Act 1971 (Britain)

Index

Note: Entries marked with an asterisk are to be found in the Glossary of drugs on p. 223.